THE 90/10 WEIGHT-LOSS PLAN

THE
90/10
WEIGHT-LOSS PLAN

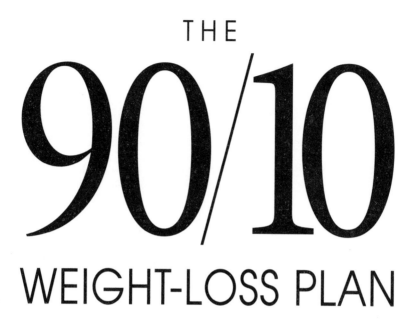

JOY BAUER, M.S., R.D., C.D.N.

RENAISSANCE BOOKS
Los Angeles

Library of Congress Control Number: 2001087571
ISBN: 1-58063-199-1

10 9 8 7 6 5 4 3 2

Published by Renaissance Books
Distributed by St. Martin's Press
Manufactured in the United States of America
First edition

To the best nourishment of all—
my husband, Ian, and children, Jesse, Cole, and Ayden Jane

ACKNOWLEDGMENTS

This book is truly the collaborative work of many people. Without their tireless support and clever contributions, it would not have happened. In fact, Lisa and Ann, your names could easily be listed on the front cover alongside mine.

To the wonderful Lisa Klugman, whose writing ability and willingness to work on such a tight deadline helped to transform my 90/10 Weight-Loss Plan into a full-blown manuscript. You have my deepest respect and gratitute.

My sincere appreciation to the world's greatest editor and now personal friend, Ann Hartley. Ann, this book is what it is because of your guidance, wisdom, and grammatical genius. You're an exceptional writer and person. I feel lucky to have had the opportunity to work with you. B₁.

To my wonderful agent, Jane Dystel. As always, you worked your magic and made things happen. Thanks also to Tracey Gardner, who kept things running smoothly.

At Renaissance Media, thanks particularly to Bill Hartley and Dick O'Connor for believing in the project and for giving me this remarkable opportunity. And my thanks to the many others at Renaissance, including Mike Dougherty, Lisa Lenthall, Jens Hussey, Kathryn Mills, Arthur Morey, Kimbria Hays, and Joe McNeely.

To the folks at St. Martin's Press, particularly Patty Rosati and Lisa Herman. Your enthusiasm and dedication are greatly appreciated.

To Eileen Livers, who was there in the very beginning. Thanks for your inspiration, encouragement, and writing expertise.

To my unstoppable (overworked/underpaid) research team: Christy Gagliano, M.S., R.D.; Tracy Bocchicchio, M.S., R.D.; Hailey

London, M.S., R.D.E.; and Tina Chen. Appreciation is an understatement! Because of all of you, we have action-packed recipes, meal plans, and Fun Foods.

To my creative cooking squad: Ellen Schloss, Carol Bauer, and Mary Malachowsky.

To the dedicated nutritionists at Joy Bauer Nutrition: Lisa Mandelbaum, M.S., R.D., C.D.N.; Lisa Young, Ph.D., R.D., C.D.N.; Jennifer Medina, M.S., R.D., C.D.E.; and Laura Pumillo, R.D., C.D.N. Thanks for your advice, opinions, and articulate information.

To Karen Robinowitz, for being an outstanding writer and for the very first mention of my book in the *New York Post*.

To David Einhorn, my legal guru and personal friend.

To Saatchi & Saatchi Advertising, particularly Judi Schipani, who successfuly organized one massive "90/10 Weight Loss Gang." To Harley Bauer and Chris Sadler, for their valuable time and expertise in production.

On a personal note, to my forever-supportive family: My husband, Ian, for his constant encouragement, patience, and amazing ability to calm me down. My extraordinary children, Jesse, Cole, and Ayden Jane. My loving parents and constant lifeline, Ellen and Artie Schloss, and Carol and Victor Bauer. My grandparents, Mary and Nat M. And to the rest of the crew: Debra, Steve, Ben, and Noah Beal; Pam and Dan Schloss; Glenn Schloss; Jason Bauer; Harley Bauer; Nancy Shapiro, Jon and Camrin Cohen; Karen Shapiro; and, of course, Cynthia Williams and Carroll Jessen.

Most importantly, a tremendous thanks to my many clients. You've enabled me to understand what works for real people. The 90/10 Plan is for you.

CONTENTS

PART THREE
Exercise, Logging, Losing—and Keeping It Off

Q: What makes you give up on a diet?

A: You can't eat what you want, so you give in to your cravings and cheat.

The big question is how to break this diet cycle. And the answer everyone's looking for is a weight-loss plan that works while still allowing you to eat the foods you love—so you'll feel satisfied and won't lose your motivation.

For the past ten years, Joy Bauer, M.S., R.D., C.D.N. has been developing just such a weight-loss plan—a plan that helps you lose weight, makes you healthier, and *even lets you eat chips, cookies, and ice cream!*

Joy Bauer is a professional nutritionist and registered dietitian, and the clients who trust and rely on her include medical and nutrition facilities, where proper diet can be as serious as a matter of life or death; Olympic athletes and celebrities who literally can't afford to be overweight; and thousands of men and women just like you who simply want to take control of their lives and be healthy and physically fit.

The 90/10 Weight-Loss Plan was designed to incorporate the majority of guidelines for sound nutrition set forth by leading scientific authorities including the U.S. Department of Agriculture, the American Dietetic Association, the American Heart Association, the American Cancer Society, and the American College of Sports Medicine.

Joy originally created the 90/10 Plan for her clients who tried to lose weight but just couldn't give up their favorite food indulgences—the Fun Foods. These clients had previously felt deprived and dissatisfied with their meals, or they felt guilty because they'd cheated. So, Joy set out to create a way of eating that was so healthy and nutritious her clients could still indulge their Fun Food fantasies—because those indulgences were actually a part of her plan.

The result of her efforts and expertise is not one of those mealtime math tests that has you checking your calculator every time you sit down at the table. The 90/10 Plan is actually a weight-loss philosophy, based on the concept that approximately 90 percent of the time you will be enjoying a balance of healthy and nutritious foods, with just enough Fun Foods to keep you happily motivated to stick with your goal.

The 90/10 Plan is calculated at three different caloric levels, so there is sure to be a level that works for your body size and personal weight-loss goal. Each level is organized on a fourteen-day cycle, with fourteen different menus for breakfast, lunch, snack, and dinner—a total of forty-two delicious and varied menus—plus a seemingly endless list of Fun Foods. There are also eleven additional main-course recipes, so you'll never get bored no matter what your desired goal.

The three levels also make the 90/10 Plan so flexible that you and your spouse, friends, coworkers, or anyone else you diet with can enjoy exactly the same meals but each at your own personalized level. It also means that when those special occasions or unusual circumstances come up you can switch from one level to another and just make a short-term adjustment to your goal.

The 90/10 Weight-Loss Plan works if you just want to lose those few stubborn pounds, it's perfect for long-term weight-loss, it's ideal for maintenance—and it's even better as a part of your everyday lifestyle.

As with any weight-loss plan, it is advised that you always check with your physician before starting something new, especially if you have a medical condition. This program was developed for the general, healthy population, therefore anyone with any medical condition will need to make special adjustments to the plan. Such adjustments are best done with the help of your personal health professional.

—Bill Hartley, Publisher

The 90/10 Weight-Loss Plan: Your Strategy for Permanent Weight Loss

CHAPTER ONE

What Do You Mean
I Can Eat Fun Foods and
Still Lose Weight?

Congratulations! You are about to change your life forever. What I'm going to tell you about the 90/10 Plan will enable you to lose weight while still eating the foods you love.

You may not believe me yet—but you will. And you'll love it. You're going to learn a weight-loss strategy that will even let you eat chocolate, cookies, chips, ice cream, and hundreds of other delicious goodies banned on other diets—and you'll still lose a significant amount of weight in just fourteen days!

I know it sounds too good to be true, but I also know it works. And it definitely is *not* a gimmick. My clients would never stand for that.

I have been a registered dietitian for more than a decade and have built one of the largest nutrition centers in New York City. I've counseled thousands of people including some of the most high-profile businessmen, celebrities, models, and Olympic athletes. Believe me, the last thing they want is another fad. They know that I've spent my entire career developing sensible nutrition plans, and they come to me because they trust me to help them improve their health, their energy, and their looks—*without* gimmicks or risky diets.

In my years of working with so many different people with such a variety of diet problems, I've become convinced that there are no protein-to-carb ratios, food-combining methods, or pill-popping regimens that will magically melt their fat away. That is why I designed the 90/10 Plan around the only time-tested principles of healthy, long-term weight loss that really work: portion control and cravings satisfaction.

The question was, how could I create a diet that would meet my clients' health needs and satisfy their taste buds at the same time? My final answer is the 90/10 Weight-Loss Plan, a scientifically designed diet that actually encourages "Fun Food" flexibility 10 percent of the time, so they'd feel satisfied throughout the weight-loss process and wouldn't feel guilty for indulging in sugary or fatty snacks.

The 90/10 Plan works for fast, effective, healthy weight loss because it includes all types of foods—nutritious items as well as fun indulgences—in a healthy balance, so that you're sure to feel satisfied and motivated. All 90/10 menus are carefully calculated to provide ample amounts of nutrition while keeping total calories low enough to guarantee weight loss.

I call it the 90/10 Plan because I recommend to my clients that about 10 percent is the average amount of calories that should come from their Fun Food choices. But, as you will see in each of the menus, there is some room for personal choice. And although my recommendation is "approximately" 10 percent, the daily menus do offer options ranging from between 100 percent of the caloric intake from healthy and nutritious food to 80 percent healthy and 20 percent fun.

But the 90/10 Plan is not about exact math anyway. It is a food philosophy for an overall weight-loss strategy. And it's a strategy that not only works for fast weight-loss but it's also, if you can believe it, even better for long-term weight maintenance!

Why? Because it teaches your mind and your body how to lose weight while learning to eat the way you should be eating for the rest of your life. The fourteen-day plan offers such a variety of delicious, nutritious meals plus treats that not only will you never feel deprived, but you'll also never get bored. And to make sure you don't, I've provided ten additional dinner recipes, so there is a total of twenty-four deliciously different main-course dinner options. That's more choices than most people who aren't on a diet would even think about.

The reason I am so confident the 90/10 Plan will work for you is that I've already seen it work for so many of my clients whom I know for a certainty lost weight and kept if off. I have also met thousands of unsuccessful dieters, and time after time I see the same pattern to their failed efforts: They have all tried to lose weight with an eating plan that is different from the way they normally eat.

Whether it is food-combination diets, high-protein diets, no-sugar diets, fat-gram-counting regimens, no-dairy/no-wheat diets, and so on, if you are not used to eating this way, you're eventually going to fall off the diet wagon. Furthermore, most leading health organizations recommend that if you're going to go on a weight-loss plan you should do it only if it's a well-rounded diet—exactly what the 90/10 Plan offers.

The 90/10 Plan is a reasonable, healthy, and easy-to-maintain approach that has already proven successful for countless dieters who found those trendy plans too restrictive and unrealistic for their lifestyles, not to mention unhealthy. And trying to follow an unreasonably difficult diet is not only unhealthy for your body but it is poisonous for your emotional health as well.

The more you jump from one diet to the next, experiencing failure after failure, the more your confidence plummets, and you learn to doubt your ability to ever successfully lose weight. It is awful to feel this way. I have heard too many painful stories from clients who have struggled with unreasonable diets and have emerged feeling more lost and hopeless than when they started. I vowed never to promote a diet that produced such frustration and heartache.

Instead, I worked to create a healthy, easy diet that would work and that was grounded in the known successful principles of weight loss—a weight-loss plan that takes as its starting point that people should lose weight eating the very same foods they dream about eating after the weight is off. That is my 90/10 Weight-Loss Plan. No gimmicks, no magic, just solid science and countless proven success stories.

As I mentioned, most of the currently trendy fad diets tend to focus on omitting entire food groups (foods your body needs, and will miss and crave) or on counting fat grams without paying attention to portion control. The 90/10 Plan focuses on what's truly important for permanent weight loss—behavioral changes that will transform your life.

On the 90/10 Plan, you will learn how to include all types of foods in your diet, and how to recognize and eat appropriate portions. The 90/10 Plan is designed to help you feel good about your ability to control and choose your food, while also making you feel good (never guilty!) about those daily fun indulgences. Because the foods you crave and enjoy are built right into the plan, balanced with more nutritious fare, you'll feel satisfied both physically and emotionally on the 90/10 Plan. Even after you've reached your weight-loss goal, you can easily incorporate the 90/10 Plan into your life on a regular basis, because everything your body needs and wants is part of the program.

In chapter 4, I will introduce you to three different caloric plans for weight loss. I will help you choose the right starting plan for you—either the 1,200-calorie plan, the 1,400-calorie plan, or the 1,600-calorie plan—based on the amount of weight you want to lose, the rate at which you would like to lose it, your dieting history, and the amount of exercise you are willing to commit to doing each week.

Once you've selected your plan, you'll have two full weeks of deliciously different daily menus to choose from. There are menus for breakfast, lunch, dinner, and snacks for each of the three plans for all fourteen days—that's forty-two meals for each plan, plus Fun Foods—which means that you don't have to spend your time obsessing over what foods do or do not fit into the 90/10 Plan and how much of them to eat.

Although controlling the number of calories you consume is important for weight loss, the 90/10 Plan is specifically designed so that you don't have to make yourself crazy counting those calories. I've already done the calorie counting for you. You'll also see that the menus are the same for the corresponding days in each of the three caloric plans, but the portion sizes or accompaniments will vary accordingly.

To limit the work required on your part, all of my food recommendations are presented in portion-controlled servings. If you don't like a particular breakfast, lunch, dinner, or snack, you can swap it for another day's menu. That's because all of the breakfasts within the specific plan you decide to follow are calorie-equivalent, all of the lunches within your particular plan are calorie-equivalent, and so are all of the dinners and snacks.

For example, if you're not a big fan of turkey burgers, you can select the dinner menu for grilled fish or linguini and red clam sauce or grilled-chicken Greek salad instead. Or, if you enjoy ordering steak when in a restaurant, you can choose the steak dinner menu in this plan. And if you want steak (or chicken, fish, or a vegetarian entrée) three nights in a row, that's okay too.

Now, about those Fun Foods. In chapter 9 you'll find an almost endless list of Fun Foods—literally hundreds of salty snacks, sweet treats, rich desserts, and other indulgences—all presented in portion-controlled servings that are precalculated to fit into each of the three caloric plans. That means each day when you see my suggestion to "enjoy a Fun Food of your choosing," your options are plentiful. And your choice of Fun Food can be enjoyed at any time of day, whatever works best for you, given your hunger level and cravings.

If you can satisfy your taste buds while dieting, you will be a successful dieter. And one of the most important ways to keep satisfied is to follow a diet that allows for variety. The 90/10 Weight-Loss

Plan does just that, with meal options ranging from omelets to waffles to pasta to red meat. Such diversity should help keep you motivated and excited about the diet and, with new and different foods to look forward to on a daily basis, you may even find yourself doing something most dieters don't get a chance to do: looking forward to lunch or dinner.

Enjoying such a wide range of foods will not only keep you satisfied but it will also help you get all of the nutrients your body needs. In fact the 90/10 meal plans are specifically designed to provide you with the most vitamins and minerals possible for the controlled amount of calories consumed.

What's more, I'll bet you'll feel more energetic and positive once you start following the 90/10 Plan. That's because, even with the inclusion of Fun Foods, the 90/10 Plan was designed to incorporate the majority of nutrition guidelines set forth by leading scientific authorities, including the American Dietetic Association, the American Heart Association, the American Cancer Society, and the American College of Sports Medicine.

Each of the three 90/10 Plans is perfectly adjusted to provide approximately 50 percent of total calories from quality carbohydrate, moderate amounts from lean protein, and limited amounts from fat—proportions that research has repeatedly proven to be optimal for good health and disease prevention.

The 90/10 menus are also low in saturated fat and dietary cholesterol, and high in fiber, phytochemicals, and antioxidants, all of which will help to reduce your risk of heart disease and certain cancers. The 90/10 Plan will also help to improve your blood circulation and increase your energy.

*   *   *

Lisa: Dieting Was All or Nothing

When Lisa, a thirty-five-year-old mother of two, came to see me she was forty-five pounds overweight. She had struggled with a weight problem her entire life, and had been on and off diets since the age of seventeen.

Over the years she had tried hundreds of diets—cabbage soup, juice fasts, big-name programs, and some of the recent trendy regimens like the high-protein/low-carbohydrate kick. Some worked, but only on a short-term basis; she always ended up gaining back the weight, sometimes more than she had lost in the first place.

When she walked into my office for the first time, Lisa felt completely frustrated and was unhappy and uncomfortable with her body. She said her energy level was so low she couldn't even play with her children (ages two and five). And she admitted that her eating habits had become out of control. She was obsessed with food and was constantly either struggling to avoid the fattening foods she loved, or bingeing on them—and, ultimately, not even enjoying her binges because she felt too guilty for eating the forbidden foods.

The main problem with Lisa's past attempts at weight loss was that all of the diet programs she tried to follow completely ruled out the fun, fattening foods that she loved and that her kids were always eating. Typically, Lisa would start off the day strong, closely following her diet-of-the-moment. But by mid-afternoon, when she was physically exhausted and emotionally drained from spending the day with her children, she would break down and start nibbling on something "off limits," usually her kids' snack foods, like Goldfish® crackers, chocolates, cookies, and the like.

Once she had gone off her diet, even slightly, Lisa would feel that she had ruined the entire day and would then proceed to eat anything and everything, thus turning a few bites of what she considered to be a "bad" food into an all-out food binge. Of course, she would always vow to start fresh again tomorrow. This would continue for a few days or weeks, until she gave up on that diet completely.

Soon enough she would attempt to stick to yet another restrictive diet plan, and the cycle would repeat itself. Lisa's "all or nothing" mentality had her bouncing between diets and eating frenzies for years, with no lasting weight-loss results.

Lisa was a perfect candidate for my 90/10 Plan. She needed to learn that all foods, including her favorite sweet and salty treats, could fit into a weight-loss plan—as long as they were eaten in portion-controlled amounts. She did not have to cut out her favorite foods or eat healthfully 100 percent of the time. More specifically, Lisa needed to plan to eat her Fun Food in the mid-afternoon while her kids were snacking, since this was the time she usually craved a treat. Feeling satisfied, and remaining confident in herself, she would then be able to continue on with a healthful dinner.

Lisa and I also discussed the importance of exercise, and we planned a realistic routine she would be able to follow. With little to no solo time, Lisa wasn't able to go to a gym to use exercise machines or to take aerobics classes. Instead, I suggested that she purchase several exercise videos and play them in her living room, also encouraging her kids to jump around with her. On other days, we determined that she could put her youngest child in the stroller and take a power walk while her older child was at school.

In just fourteen days, Lisa had lost seven pounds. After two and a half months, she was twenty pounds thinner, and looked and felt fabulous. Two years later, all the extra weight plus an additional two pounds is off. Even more important, Lisa no longer views foods as "good" or "bad." Instead, she continues to follow the 90/10 Plan, eating healthy foods 90 percent of the time while satisfying her cravings for Fun Foods 10 percent of the time. With the 90/10 Weight-Loss Plan, Lisa lost weight, learned healthy yet nonrestrictive eating habits, and changed her life.

Of course, not everyone who wants to lose weight is like Lisa, with her long history of dieting. You may have started dieting only recently, in an effort to lose those pounds that inevitably creep on after age thirty.

By that time most people's eating habits are well ingrained and may seem impossible to change. After all, once you have been eating a certain way for so many years without needing to diet, changing your eating habits can seem like an overwhelming effort. But, as my clients prove to me again and again, even the most stubborn or busy or set-in-their-ways people can learn to follow the 90/10 Plan.

They can do this because the 90/10 Weight-Loss Plan satisfies rather than deprives, and can be adapted to fit anyone's lifestyle. Best of all, the 90/10 Plan is usually not so drastically different from the way most people have been eating all along.

*   *   *

Steven: Diets Didn't Fit His Lifestyle

Another client, Steven, a fifty-year-old businessman, never had a weight problem until he hit forty. Between forty and fifty, though,

Steven gained twenty pounds, which left him feeling heavy, sluggish, unattractive, and uncomfortable in his clothing.

The weight gain had also caused Steven's cholesterol level to shoot up over 260 (a healthy cholesterol level for a middle-aged man is anywhere under 200), and he developed serious high blood pressure. He had even been put on a blood-pressure-lowering medication. His cardiologist had been nagging Steven to lose weight and to eat healthier in order to bring his numbers down to an acceptable level.

Steven tried several diets, including a vegetarian diet, a high-protein/low-carbohydrate plan, and several of his own approaches, such as skipping breakfast and lunch so that he could indulge at dinner when he often had to entertain clients at restaurants.

With each diet attempt, Steven would lose a few pounds, typically two to five in just one week, but the diet didn't last long. None of the plans he tried were realistic for his lifestyle, and so he would be forced to go off them quickly. And as soon as he tried to eat normally again, the numbers on the scale would rise, often leaving him heavier than he had been before he started the last diet.

Before our first visit, I had asked Steven to keep a food diary. Looking at it, I saw that Steven's food choices during the day were typically high-carbohydrate and often high-fat, and severely lacking in protein. He would start the day with a ritualistic mug of coffee, flavored with sugar and cream, then opt for a corn muffin or a bagel with cream cheese, along with orange juice, for lunch.

No wonder he complained of afternoon headaches and fatigue— he was probably suffering bouts of hypoglycemia from low blood sugar because, for his size, he didn't eat enough protein and was taking in too much refined carbohydrate and fat.

And his restaurant dinners were outright dangerous for him. After eating virtually nothing satisfying or nutritious all day, he was ravenous by dinner and would often reach right for the bread basket at restaurants, then later go on to order dessert. A typical dinner for Steven consisted of three alcoholic drinks, four slices of bread with butter, a large steak, a baked potato with sour cream and butter, creamed spinach, and a piece of cake. And again he had cream and sugar in his coffee.

I understood why Steven made the food choices he did during the day—they were easy, fast, and required little thought. With his busy work schedule, he doesn't have the time or energy to plan elaborate meals, nor does he care to do so. But there are plenty of equally accessible breakfast and lunch foods that are loaded with nutrition, low in calories and fat, and that would leave him feeling much better, more energetic, and less ravenous at dinnertime.

Steven obviously needed some leeway with dinner. I didn't expect him to be able to go out for dinner and keep his fingers out of the bread basket all the time, or to give up desserts for good, or even to cut out alcohol (although I encouraged him to limit his alcoholic drinks to one per day). The 90/10 Plan could help him eat smarter and feel more satisfied during the day so that dinners out would no longer be such high-calorie, high-fat, supersized meals.

Together, Steven and I planned out hearty, well-balanced breakfasts and lunches that were appealing to him and that were also easy and effortless. For example, he could opt for fruit and yogurt for breakfast, a salad and soup or a salad and sandwich for lunch. It was easy for Steven to see—and feel—that a turkey sandwich on whole-wheat bread with lettuce, tomato, and two slices of cheese, plus a side salad, for lunch was much more filling than his previous choice of a corn muffin and a glass of orange juice.

The new meal was also ten times more nutritious and, because it provided more protein and fiber, it helped to stabilize his blood-sugar levels, boost his energy, and relieve his afternoon headaches. To take off the hunger-edge and to further guard against Steven feeling overly hungry at dinnertime, we agreed that an afternoon snack was also in order. But we made that snack a healthy, low-calorie one so that Steven could indulge in his Fun Food at dinner, when he was most apt to crave it.

For Steven, that Fun Food might be strawberries and whipped cream, a scoop of vanilla ice cream with hot fudge, a small piece of chocolate cake, or even a few extra slices of bread. He could also consider using his Fun Food allowance as two glasses of wine with dinner.

His entrée could remain a moderate-size steak, although I did encourage him to alternate with a piece of grilled chicken or fish in order to bring down his elevated cholesterol numbers. I also had Steven substitute his usual fat-laden creamed spinach and sour-cream–filled baked potato with a salad and plenty of steamed vegetables. And, of course, skim milk in his coffee versus the cream and sugar.

What surprised Steven the most was that even with all the satisfying foods to choose from each day, I had carefully calculated his meals so that he was eating only 1,600 calories a day, which was guaranteed to result in weight loss for him. Following the 90/10 Plan, Steven didn't have to give up all the foods that he loved, which helped motivate him to stick to the plan.

Right away he felt less irritable, more energetic, and more productive at work. He was not starving by dinner, didn't feel deprived while dining at restaurants, and knocked off the weight in no time. In fact Steven lost ten pounds in just fourteen days and watched more weight come off over the following weeks. Four years later, the weight is still off.

Not only that but his cholesterol level is down from 260 to 173, and his blood pressure has decreased enough to please his doctor and get him off medication. It helped that I convinced Steven to take the stairs at work and to park half a mile from his office, so that he would be forced to squeeze at least a little physical activity into each day (not bad for someone who swore he had no time to exercise).

Although Steven isn't getting the amount of exercise I typically recommend, he is burning more calories than usual, and the physical activity has helped him develop the positive mindset to support his healthful food choices during the day.

While exercise is an important part of any weight-loss and weight-management program, even people who exercise regularly may have difficulty losing weight if their eating habits are fighting their weight-loss efforts.

For example, these days Americans are obsessed with cutting fat from their diets because they believe that is the key to weight loss. Fat-free and low-fat food products are all the rage, but such items are not the weight-loss magic bullets they seem to be. Granted, for the most part the explosion of lower-fat foods on the market has been a wonderful tool, enabling people to painlessly lower their cholesterol intake and total fat intake. But for many people the words *fat-free* or *low-fat* are an invitation to overeat those foods.

The problem: Just because a product is fat-free doesn't mean it's calorie-free. And many fat-free foods can pack in just as many calories as their original fat-containing counterparts. In the end, excessive calories—no matter where they come from, be it from fat, carbohydrate, or protein—will result in weight gain, or in the prevention of weight loss.

*   *   *

Marcy: Her Diet Was Actually Too Low in Fat

When Marcy, a single, twenty-seven-year-old advertising executive, came to see me, she was struggling to lose seven to ten pounds. An avid exerciser, she couldn't understand why she didn't lose the weight, especially because she was careful to eat a low-fat diet.

Marcy's weight problem started in college when, during her first year, she gained the typical "Freshman 15" from all the late-night pizzas and study-session snacking. At twenty-five she finally made an effort to lose the unwanted weight.

Marcy began working out four to five times a week at the gym and followed a low-fat diet. She even read food labels and counted fat grams. The first five pounds dropped off within a month, but then the scale stopped moving. Despite almost two years' worth of effort, she was unable to knock off the last seven to ten pounds.

When I learned the details of Marcy's daily diet, I wasn't surprised that she was having difficulty losing weight. To replace the fat in her diet, she was overcompensating with low-fat and fat-free products. Her diet was actually too low in fat, which no doubt left her feeling hungry and dissatisfied, and much more apt to reach for carbohydrates and to overeat them. Plus, the number of calories she was getting from carbohydrate and protein sources was higher than she was able to burn off during her workouts. Her diet was loaded with fruit, bread, pasta, pretzels, fat-free cookies, frozen yogurt, and fat-free jellybeans and gummy bears.

Marcy confessed that she wouldn't go near "real desserts" due to the fat phobia she had developed over the years, but never hesitated to treat herself to large portions of fat-free versions. When I showed her the calorie comparison of one regular cookie with 4 grams of fat (75 calories) versus the ten nonfat cookies (500 calories) she sometimes ate during the course of one day, Marcy was shocked.

The 90/10 Plan, with its balance of carbohydrate, fat, and protein, plus its inclusion of Fun Foods, was perfect for Marcy. Following the 90/10 Plan, she felt more satisfied after her meals and snacks, and no longer felt the need to overeat fat-free and low-fat substitutions. Marcy was thrilled to be able to indulge again in ice cream and cookies. She admitted that she had forgotten how good the "real stuff" tasted, and that because of the taste and because she knew she was eating the full-fat, satisfying version, one serving was plenty.

After fourteen days of following the 90/10 Plan and continuing with her exercise regimen, Marcy lost five pounds. She was thrilled, especially since she hadn't seen the scale move in two years. She lost a total of ten pounds by week eight. A year and a half later, Marcy is still eating according to the 90/10 Plan and the weight is still off. She no longer overeats fat-free muffins and low-fat cookies, but she does regularly enjoy two of her childhood favorites—peanut butter and m&m®s.

The success my clients have had with the 90/10 Weight-Loss Plan has proven to them and confirmed to me that many of today's best-known diet gurus are wrong. The truth is that all foods can fit into a weight-loss and weight-management program, even foods high in sugar, starch, and fat.

And that's not the only diet myth I happily debunk based on what I've learned from real experience with real people. I've devoted an entire chapter to answering the most common questions my clients ask, questions such as, "Does the timing of my meals matter?" and "Are there certain food combinations that will help me burn calories more efficiently?" You will be amazed to learn the truths about some of the food and diet myths: that not only do they not work, but that they can also actually impair weight-loss and weight-management efforts.

My clients and I also worked out methods, based on the individual's personal healthy weight range, that will help you to determine how much weight you should plan to lose on the 90/10 Plan. And, because it proved so helpful for most people to keep track of their food intake and exercise, I developed the food logs you'll find in chapter 11. You'll be surprised how these food logs can help you to evaluate your personal eating patterns and solve some of the dieting problems that have kept you from success in the past.

As I said at the beginning, the 90/10 Plan was inspired by what I learned from working with clients for more than ten years in my nutrition practice. It was a lesson in basic human nature at work: If you tell someone no, you must not eat this or that, it only makes their urge for those particular foods stronger. But if a client's weight-loss program was very close to the way that person should be eating permanently, for the rest of their life, they were more successful at keeping the weight off.

That meant that the first step was to design a diet that didn't omit entire food groups or deprive dieters of their favorite foods. And, as you've probably guessed from the number of times I've mentioned the words *health* and *nutrition,* it was just as important to me that any diet I designed would incorporate the guidelines of the major health organizations, my own nutritional schooling, and the advice of top doctors whom I respect.

The happy result is the 90/10 Weight-Loss Plan—a diet that includes all foods in moderation, with room for your favorite snacks. So you *can* continue to eat your favorite jellybeans, chips, candy bars, or ice cream, and the best part is you now know that when you do, you are actually helping yourself shed pounds.

*   *   *

William: A Smoking Success

A fifty-six-year-old close family friend, William, had been carrying an extra thirty to forty pounds for the past twenty years, ever since he quit smoking cigarettes. Basically he went from being a skinny man addicted to nicotine to an overweight man addicted to sugar.

"I never was a good eater," remembers William. "I rarely touched a vegetable or fruit, and I ate too much red meat and quite a bit of candy. I never even tried to lose all the weight I gained after I quit smoking, because it seemed like too much work. I'd listen to friends and coworkers talk about different diets, and it didn't seem like an enjoyable hobby. So I passed on the whole diet-and-weight-loss option and just decided to remain overweight."

He would give healthy eating a try for a couple of days or a couple of hours and then sink right back into his old, comfy eating habits. He just wasn't motivated.

I found it difficult to watch William's questionable food choices and not say anything to him, especially when we ate meals together so often, but unless someone asks for help, offering it unsolicited will only make them feel uncomfortable. Losing weight and making healthier lifestyle changes are purely personal commitments that work only when a person is *ready* to commit.

However, because he understood my genuine concern, and without actually nagging him, I was finally able to convince William to give the 90/10 Weight-Loss Plan a shot. I promised him that it would be easy, that it would satisfy him, and, most important, that he could continue to eat his donuts, butterscotch candies, and Chuckles®.

I also had the support of his thin wife, Carol. She and their three sons had been nagging William to lose weight for twenty years. Carol was concerned about his high cholesterol levels, hypertension, and a bad back—all primarily due to the extra weight. He also had a history of gallbladder attacks, which had led to the removal of his gallbladder.

"I'll admit that being in pain due to my back and having to just rest in bed for a week also made me want to lose weight, but I didn't feel like sticking to a diet until Joy promised that the 90/10 Plan would include all my usual foods, specifically Mallomars® cookies," says William. "When I saw that I could still eat my Chuckles®, cookies, and other sweets, I figured I could give it a try. So I called Joy and asked if she could schedule some office time with me that week to go over her 90/10 Weight-Loss Plan."

I was so delighted! I scheduled time for him to come into the office the very next day. I placed him on the 1,600-calorie plan so that he would feel very comfortable and satisfied. We went over the meals together. He liked eight of the fourteen breakfasts and felt that he could manage five of the fourteen lunches. Miraculously, William liked almost all of the dinner options, with the exception of a few. Because he is a successful businessman and dinner with clients is a frequent affair, he committed to either the steak meal or the steamed Chinese meal when eating out. At home, his very eager wife helped him along every step of the way. Thank you, Carol!

Due to his bad back, we didn't start things off with exercise, and, fortunately, found that we didn't need to—after two weeks, William had lost ten-and-a-half pounds. Sometime later, with more pounds off and his back feeling slightly better, he began seeing a physical therapist, doing stretches and strengthening work.

William's entire family and circle of friends, including myself, were elated to see the positive effects of his weight loss. He seemed to grow younger and more vibrant with every week that passed. His added vigor made him become more interested in his eating and fitness in general. He started keeping articulate food logs and actually asked me to look them over every week. He even faxed the logs to my office when he was out of town. What's more, he bought a few nutrition books and even subscribed to a health magazine. Amazing!

Three and a half months after starting the 90/10 Plan, William had lost a total of thirty pounds, which was our goal.

"I'm confident that my weight loss is permanent, because I've learned, finally, how to eat healthy," says William. "It's really not as difficult as I imagined it would be. I didn't have to give up any of my favorite foods. I have learned that if I eat healthfully the majority of the time, I can have flexibility for fun indulgences. Best of all, I feel really great. My back pain is markedly better and I move easier. I would recommend the 90/10 Plan to anyone who loves to eat and hates to diet."

CHAPTER TWO

Your Diet Questions Answered

I have never met anyone who didn't have a question about dieting and weight loss. Many nutrition experts claim to possess the magic solution, whether it be a high-protein/low-carb diet, a fat-free regimen, juice-fasting, a "detoxification" plan, or food combining. There are weight-loss books that feature diets for different blood types, body types—even for different personality types.

Unfortunately, though magic solutions to weighty woes are extremely enticing, the nutritional logic behind these new-and-different dieting techniques is often far from valid and is unrealistic for the long haul.

Yet new diets continue to flourish, despite their lack of clinical trials and data. Weight-loss foods, drugs, and herbs are being manufactured constantly, including meal-replacement shakes and fat-burning pills, and the airwaves are filled with infomercials promoting products that promise to change your body forever, with only a few monthly bites on your credit card. Some of these weight-loss methods do nothing more than leave you weighing the same, while other diet scams can actually harm your physical and mental health.

Counting calories is stressful. Labeling foods "good" and "bad" can be nerve-racking. Getting excited about one diet plan after the other is extremely self-defeating and discouraging. No wonder so many people have such a hard time losing weight! The weight-loss industry is chock-full of myths and misconceptions. Everyone has something to say on the matter. The real problem is that there is so much information out there—most of which is confusing or contradictory—that most of us aren't quite sure about what we should be doing.

The good news is that dieting doesn't have to be so hard. And eating healthy to lose weight does not have to leave you feeling deprived or hungry. In fact, you can enjoy it—eating healthy can (gasp) even be fun. You just have to know the facts, the nutritional values, and your body's basic needs.

Who doesn't love to eat? Who doesn't crave treats that most diets label "forbidden"? Eating is one of life's greatest pleasures! The 90/10 Weight-Loss Plan combines this healthy spirit of food celebration with solid, factual, well-balanced nutrition.

But before I explain the plan in detail, let's review the most popular dieting myths and get some important facts straight.

WHAT TO EXPECT

How Much Weight Will I Lose on the 90/10 Plan?

On average, you'll lose up to ten pounds in the first two weeks. You should always expect to lose more weight in the beginning. The exact amount you'll lose depends on how many pounds you have to shed and how much you're eating before you start the plan. Those who have many pounds to shed, and those who were eating large quantities beforehand, will most likely lose more.

You should expect to lose water weight in the beginning, because food tends to hold water. Once you cut back on the amount of calories that you consume, your body will be holding on to less water and you will immediately feel lighter and less bloated. Within a week the scale should register a loss of a few pounds, which should be wonderfully uplifting and a great incentive to keep going.

Ladies, if you follow the plan with your boyfriend or husband, don't be upset if he loses more weight than you do. Clinical studies show that men lose more weight than women lose when following the same eating plan. The reason for this unfair reality? Men tend to eat greater volumes of food than women eat on a day-to-day basis, so to follow the same diet plan men must reduce their meals by a larger percentage. Also, men are often bigger and therefore burn more calories.

Don't plan on losing up to ten pounds *every* two weeks. After the first two weeks, your weight loss should balance out to between a half-pound and two pounds a week. If you find that you're losing more, you'll need to move to the next caloric level within the plan.

Losing weight too quickly will leave you dehydrated and tired. Or, even worse, you'll lose muscle, also known as "lean body mass." The more muscle you have, the higher your metabolism—at rest, muscle burns significantly more calories than fat. Restricting your calories too much will force your body to burn muscle for energy and you'll have a hard time keeping those pounds off.

Remember: The way to effectively lose weight for the long term is to preserve your lean body mass while decreasing body fat.

Will Carbohydrates Make Me Fat?

In this era of trendy low-carb and no-carb diets, this may be the best thing you've heard since 1992: Carbohydrates will *not* make you fat. In fact carbohydrates, and especially quality carbohydrates eaten in moderation, will improve your health while making you look leaner and feel more energized. Carbohydrates are the body's preferred source of energy. Some of the body's tissues—red blood cells and some parts of the brain, for instance—can *only* use carbohydrates as fuel.

Picking and choosing the kind of carbohydrates you eat, however, is key. Excellent, high-quality, carbohydrate-rich foods include fruits, vegetables, and whole grains. In the whole-grain category, look for whole-grain breads, whole-grain breakfast cereals, brown rice, oatmeal, wheat germ, kasha, bulgar, couscous, bran, wheat bran, wheat berries, quinoa, barley, and popcorn. You can also pick up whole-grain pastas, crackers, and chips at your local grocery store. Just read those labels! Your healthy goal is to limit refined carbohydrates and simple sugars (like candy, jam, jelly, white rice) and anything made with white flour (like white-flour bread, pancakes, and crackers).

Important weight-loss fact: Although green leafy vegetables and bulgar wheat are healthier carbohydrates to consume than a bagel with strawberry jam, the calories are the same. All carbohydrates, regardless of quality, supply 4 calories per gram of carbohydrate. Choosing quality carbs over low-quality carbs is simply a matter of better nutrition, which will give you greater resistance to illness and increased long-term energy. Whole grains, fruits, and vegetables all provide vitamins, minerals, fiber, and phytochemicals, which are powerful plant substances that can help fight off disease and promote longevity.

As luck would have it, most humans with functioning taste buds have at least one favorite food (or two, or three, or eighteen) that falls into the less-than-stellar, white-flour/refined-sugar carbohydrate category. And that's fine! The 90/10 Plan recognizes our undying passion for pizza, cookies, and chocolate. Do any of us really want to go through life without these tasty treats? I think not! When we label white-flour carbs as "off limits," "cheating," or "bad," those carbs immediately seem even more attractive.

Some people don't think too much about their favorite treats until they start a diet that considers those treats as going "off." Then they resist and resist and resist some more, until they fall off the wagon, landing smack in the middle of more bagels and potato chips than they would have ever wanted, if only the dangerous *forbidden* word had never been used.

Then dieting's number-one worst enemy sets in—guilt. They feel guilty for indulging. They lose faith in their ability to ever successfully follow a diet to reach their goal weight. All this heartache, just because their weight-loss plan didn't leave room for their favorite treats.

The 90/10 Plan avoids this very common dieting syndrome by making room for some refined carbohydrates, such as cookies and candy. All these soul-soothing extras are featured in carefully calculated and controlled portions, so that the bulk of your calories comes from quality, nutritious foods. Remember, the 90/10 Plan is about celebrating the joy of food while you lose weight and get healthy. If you don't go easy on yourself, and work to satisfy your (natural) passion for dessert and other munchies, then sticking to a plan for the long term is going to be difficult, if not impossible.

One final warning: Diets completely lacking in carbohydrate can be extremely dangerous. When the body is deprived of carbohydrate, it is forced to use protein to make glucose (also known as blood sugar; it is the fuel that our cells need to survive).

Forcing your body to do this inhibits its ability to make proper, optimum use of the protein you do eat. Its first priority then becomes creating adequate glucose, while a few crucial bodily functions become secondary in importance, including the digestion of fat. Impairing fat metabolism means that the fat in your diet is only partially broken down, which results in your body's production of ketones. This condition is called ketosis and it can alter the normal acid-base balance of the body, which tends to cause dizziness, fatigue, chronic bad breath, and, in some cases, serious illness.

Diets that feature unlimited protein cause another unpleasant side-effect: constipation. Quality fiber is found in the kind of whole grains, fruits, and vegetables that are often avoided on high-protein food plans. Carbohydrates supply fiber, and fiber promotes bowel regularity, which reduces the risk of hemorrhoids, diverticulosis, and irritable bowel syndrome, while lowering cholesterol and stabilizing blood-sugar levels.

An excessive intake of protein over an extended period of time will have negative effects on your entire system. Protein also interferes with your body's absorption of calcium, and that increases your chances of osteoporosis—a disorder that especially affects women. Eating *only* turkey, chicken, tofu, fish, or eggs does far more harm than good, even if you reap a temporary weight loss from that sort of diet. The key to successfully losing weight—and keeping it off—is balance, moderation, and satisfaction, which is exactly what the 90/10 Weight-Loss Plan is all about.

It is the total number of calories you consume that determines weight gain or weight loss, not any "magic" ratio of protein, carbs, and fats; a balance of those is required for optimum health and maximum pleasure, not for weight loss.

Remember this simple, commonsense fact: If you eat more calories than you burn, you'll gain weight; if you burn more calories than you eat, you'll lose weight. For example, if you eat 3,000 calories' worth of apples, and you burn less than 3,000 calories, you'll gain weight. This is also true if you had consumed 3,000 calories' worth of cookies or 3,000 calories' worth of chicken—if you don't burn up all those calories, you will gain weight. Unlimited portions of any food will likely cause weight gain, whether it's candy, meat, dairy, or anything else.

Does the Timing of My Meals Really Matter?
Yes and no.

Yes, because you want to keep your appetite satiated throughout the day. When you spend your mornings and afternoons eating very little, it can backfire. You may feel fine throughout the day, but by seven o'clock in the evening you feel ravenous. And we all know what that leads to . . . uncontrollable overeating!

Eating regularly throughout the day provides your body with constant fuel, which kills your urge to binge. Your blood-sugar levels (blood glucose) remain in equilibrium. Your desire for munchies is kept on an even keel. If you don't eat for a long time, you may suffer from a hypoglycemic episode, which results from lowered blood-sugar levels and produces such not-fun symptoms as headache, moodiness, dizziness, irritability, and fatigue.

And *no*, because calories affect the body in the exact same way no matter what time you eat them.

Many diet plans advise people not to eat after a certain time in the evening. This might be good advice, but not because late-night eating will necessarily cause you to gain weight. Controlling your eating after dinner is a smart idea because evenings are when most people attempt to rid themselves from the stress of the day—via overeating. Food, as we know, can be a wonderful distraction, tension-buster, hobby, and mood-lifter.

So be aware of your tendency to use food to soothe your nerves, especially after dinner. Sitting at home, reading magazines or watching television, is when most of us tend to overeat. In fact recent studies have shown that nighttime eaters wind up eating more collective calories than people who do not eat after dinner. Of course, if you are truly hungry at night you should eat something, because hunger can interfere with sleep. Don't allow any time guidelines to cause you to feel guilty if you really need the food. And if you find that you're feeling most munchy in the evening, you may decide to have your Fun Food after dinner. Just be sure to keep tight control on your portions.

The timing of your meals will not affect your progress. But skipping breakfast or lunch, or waiting too long between meals, will zap your energy, dampen your mood, and increase your chances of overdoing the calories or making poor food choices later.

Remember, though, it is only the total number of calories consumed that causes weight gain or weight loss.

Are There Certain Food Combinations That Will Help Me Burn Calories More Efficiently?

No, food combining (eating protein and carbohydrate separately, at different meals) will not affect your body's ability to burn calories.

Despite the popularity of food-combining diets, there is no specific scientific evidence to suggest that carbohydrate or protein is more easily digested when eaten alone. Or that food combining increases metabolism or helps the weight-loss process in any way. You won't lose weight quicker on a food-combining diet, but you will have to resist many healthy, popular meals—like a basic tuna sandwich!

The body produces specific enzymes to break down food. In healthy individuals, these enzymes are produced in response to all foods. There are specific enzymes that break down fat, specific enzymes that break down carbohydrate, and specific enzymes that break down protein.

The concept behind food combining states that the enzymes that break down protein work more efficiently if they are not burdened by the presence of the enzymes that break down carbohydrate. Yet eating a protein-only meal will not negate the presence of the carb enzymes or fat enzymes. In fact there are few foods that contain only protein without a trace of fat—and even fewer foods that contain only carbohydrate without a trace of protein.

Notice the nutrition labels on your favorite foods. Although some foods will be predominant in one macronutrient (protein, carbohydrate, or fat), most often you'll see traces of the other macronutrients in the mix as well. Food combining will not inhibit, nor will it enhance, your body's ability to digest carbs, proteins, and fats.

There are, however, certain food combinations that help the body absorb vitamins and minerals. For example, foods loaded with vitamin C are a healthy companion to iron-rich foods, because vitamin C enhances the body's ability to absorb iron. Vitamin D helps our bodies absorb calcium, which is why milk manufacturers add vitamin D to milk.

In order for a weight-loss plan to work, it should meet two standards. First, it should benefit health and increase energy levels, and second, it should satisfy your natural desire for tasty, normal meals. By offering a nice mix of carbohydrate, protein, and fat at each meal, the 90/10 Weight-Loss Plan meets both criteria.

Do Herbal Remedies or Over-the-Counter "Dietary" Supplements Promote Weight Loss?

The shelves of many health food stores are filled with herbal remedies and dietary supplements that claim to promote weight loss or offer a quick metabolism boost. These products come in many forms: pills, powders, shakes, candy bars, and even diet teas.

And though it's true that some herbal remedies may be very helpful in treating many different ailments, including depression, motion sickness, anxiety, and insomnia, as far as weight loss goes, there is no magic remedy. In reality, much of the unchecked research touting herbs and dietary supplements for weight loss has studied individuals who took the supplement in question while following calorie-restricted diets and/or rigorous exercise programs.

It is therefore not possible to determine whether the supplement affected the individuals' weight loss, or whether the weight loss was simply a natural result of diet and/or exercise.

Furthermore, herbal and dietary supplement manufacturers do not need to register with the FDA (Food and Drug Administration) nor get FDA approval before producing or selling dietary supplements (unlike prescription and over-the-counter medicines). Therefore, some over-the-counter weight-loss potions are more than a waste of money—they can be dangerous. Some herbs may even interfere with prescription medications and may lead to serious side effects. If you're interested in investigating herbal weight-loss remedies and other dietary supplements, I strongly suggest you talk to your physician first.

Here is the lowdown on some herbs and dietary supplements that are sold to encourage weight loss and improve health:

Ma Huang, Also Known as Ephedra: Although there are many ingredients in popular herbal concoctions that may lead to health problems, this substance is especially dangerous. It has been known to promote weight loss, but ingesting it puts your body at great risk. Taking Ma Huang can produce effects that are very much like taking speed, or amphetamines. It can increase heart rate and raise blood pressure, which may ultimately lead to heart palpitations, tremors, headaches, dizziness, and insomnia. All of these complications are anxiety-provoking and stressful on the body. For individuals who suffer from hypertension or heart conditions, Ma Huang can be lethal. (And it is quite possible for someone to have a heart condition and not even know it.)

Spirulina: It was once thought that spirulina could suppress appetite by increasing levels of the amino acid, phenylalanine. However, human studies using this blue-green algae are limited, and there is no data to support its effectiveness in weight loss. Also, spirulina can accumulate heavy metals from contaminated water, and some people have been found to have allergic reactions to this supplement. I do not recommend it.

Chromium Picolinate: Although quite a few studies have been conducted, this supplement has yet to be linked to weight loss. The good news: taken in moderation, there are no major side effects. It is important to understand, however, that excessive intake can lead to toxic levels of chromium in the body. There is also no need to take supplements, as a balanced diet offers adequate levels of chromium.

Pyruvate: Studies on pyruvate have not warranted serious medical consideration. It is not clear whether the individuals in the studies lost weight because of the supplement itself or because they simultaneously decreased their caloric intake and/or increased their exercise regimes. In addition, this substance tends to cause gas and diarrhea.

Carnitine: Our bodies naturally produce a small concentration of carnitine and the rest of what we need comes from the food we eat. Excess amounts are completely unnecessary, a waste of money, and can be potentially toxic.

Co-enzyme Q10: Like the rest of these supplements and herbs, co-enzyme Q10 hasn't been scientifically proven to stimulate weight loss.

The following three herbal remedies should be avoided, because they have been linked to specific health problems:

Comfrey: This has been proven to cause liver damage.

Lobelia: Breathing problems, rapid heart rate, sweating, coma, and death have sometimes been caused by lobelia.

Yohimbe: This may cause nervous disorders, paralysis, fatigue, stomach problems, and death.

Why Do Some People Gain Weight Easily While Others Do Not?

There is not one single, simple reason but a variety of factors that influence an individual's tendency to lose or gain weight. There are, in fact, five major factors that can affect your own unique dieting and weight-loss profile:

Constant Dieting: Yo-yo dieting can lower your metabolism, which ultimately leads to weight gain and difficulty in losing weight.

Inactivity: Weight gain may also be caused by a lower metabolism. It is a proven, indisputable fact that exercise increases your metabolism and influences weight loss. Exercise also increases lean body mass, which in turn increases your metabolic rate.

The psychological benefits of exercise are also not to be taken lightly. Exercise has a positive mental effect. It can make you feel happier, increase your self-esteem, and give you a feeling of can-do optimism. A regular exercise program will not only help your body burn off fat, but it will also help you maintain confidence. Exercise will help you believe in your ability to achieve what you set out to do—including eating a healthy diet, reaching your weight goal, and maintaining it with style, good humor, and a relaxed, happy attitude.

Genetics: Inherited body types, body shapes, and build account for some of the differences among individuals. (It would be a pretty boring world if there weren't any of these differences!) A family history of obesity increases, up to 50 percent, your chances of becoming obese.

Please, don't let these odds discourage you one iota! Though genes may make you more susceptible to gaining weight, you can absolutely overcome your genetic makeup. Diet, exercise, and conscious lifestyle changes can keep your weight down and your body looking and feeling fit. Just because your parents or family may be overweight, doesn't necessarily mean that you have "fat genes"; you may just have relations with "fat habits." Your family members may be overweight due to lavish eating styles and/or lack of exercise, not due to genetic makeup.

Gender: Also impacts your weight. Women's bodies are predisposed to carrying more fat than are men's bodies, which no amount of feminism or women's-rights rallying is ever going to change—or there would probably be ten thousand women marching in Washington tomorrow! Adult men usually have 10 to 20 percent more muscle—and less body fat—than women of the same age and weight. (I know, ladies, it stinks!)

Because muscle burns more calories than fat, men are automatically more predisposed to losing weight more easily than women are. Men are also more likely to maintain their weight while eating more food, whereas women's bodies aim to store fat for pregnancy and breastfeeding. This is also what makes women's bodies beautifully curvaceous.

Temperature: Believe it or not, this is an issue. Your metabolism is slightly higher when the climate is brutally cold or unbearably hot. This is because your body and metabolism need to be more active to help keep you healthy and comfortable at extreme temperatures.

Now, no one likes being so cold that they shiver and their teeth chatter, but look on the bright side: Shivering keeps you warm and burns calories. I wouldn't suggest job hunting at the North Pole, but these cold-weather realities may change your opinion of the bitter winter season. Similarly, when the weather is very hot, your metabolism increases to help keep your body cool. Given these options, migrating to the Tropics sounds like the better extreme.

Present Body Weight: Your present weight will influence how much weight you are likely to lose, and how quickly. Those who are very overweight can lose large amounts in the first couple of months, in part because the more you weigh, the more calories your body will burn. It takes a considerable amount of effort and energy for a three-hundred-pound person to walk one mile—after all, they must carry three hundred pounds the entire distance.

Medical Disorders: These can affect your ability to lose weight. If you suspect you're gaining weight in spite of a moderate diet and regular exercise program, or if you're having a very difficult time losing weight, get a full medical checkup. A surprising number of people suffer from conditions such as thyroid disease, which has an enormous effect on metabolism and weight. You could have a hypothyroid, which is an underactive thyroid and is actually quite common. A healthy thyroid releases hormones that control your metabolism and boost energy levels. A dysfunctional thyroid may produce an inadequate amount of hormones, which slows your metabolic rate, makes you feel sluggish, and often leads to weight gain. Hypothyroid can be detected with a simple blood test and is completely treatable with medication. Be aware of your body. Like "walking pneumonia," you can easily have hypothyroidism and not even know it.

Should I Use Artificial Sweeteners and Diet Sodas?

This is a personal decision. Some dieters choose to avoid them completely, some use them regularly, and others prefer to use them in moderation. For the record, I am not a fan of artificial sweeteners. However, the American Dietetic Association (ADA) remains neutral.

On the 90/10 Weight-Loss Plan, the option is yours. You may choose to drink diet beverages and sweeten your food with artificial sweeteners in moderation.

Will I Lose More Weight If I Omit Fat from My Diet?

No. Depriving your body of fat is unhealthy. Plus, consuming fat-free meal after fat-free meal has been shown to eradicate all traces of humor from the personality . . .

However, like the war on carbs, the fat-quotient question has caused many heated debates. Different "experts" say different things. There are constant contradictions. Some weight-loss diets feature unlimited fat, while others keep your fat intake as close to zero as possible. The healthy person's answer to the fat-quotient question lies somewhere between these two extremes.

The American Dietetic Association, the American Cancer Society, the American College of Sports Medicine, and the American Heart Association all agree on how much fat we should consume for optimum health. All these prestigious, regulated, and well-respected institutions say a healthy diet should be comprised of less than 30 percent fat coming from your total daily calories. *Limited* but not *eliminated.*

Controlling your fat intake will promote weight loss because ounce-for-ounce, gram-per-gram, fat has more calories than does carbohydrate or protein. In fact carbohydrate and protein both supply only 4 calories per gram, while one gram of fat contains more than double: 9 calories per gram. Clearly, fat packs a calorie-filled wallop and will easily cause weight gain when eaten in excess.

Completely omitting all fat from your diet is unnecessary, unpalatable, and, most of all, dangerous. Always remember: A diet will never be successful if you're unhappy with what you eat. If you don't treat your taste buds to a bit of delicious fat, you'll be miserable . . . and will most likely experience the common condition of rebellious overeating at a later date.

What's the Story with Healthy and Unhealthy Fats?

The healthy fats, monounsaturated and polyunsaturated, are necessary for energy, a strong immune system, a healthy heart, good moods, and bowel regularity. The good fats promote glowing skin and shiny hair, and are required for insulating and protecting our vital organs. Also, both monounsaturated and polyunsaturated fats taste good! They help you feel satisfied and help keep the appetite under control.

Foods rich in monounsaturated fats include avocados, olive oil, canola oil, and peanuts. Polyunsaturated fats can be found in corn oil, safflower oil, sunflower oil, and soybean oil. Certain polyunsaturated fats, called omega-3 fatty acids, have been linked to lower incidences of cancer and heart disease. Omega-3 fatty acids are found in fatty fish (such as salmon, mackerel, tuna, trout, and sardines), flaxseeds, and walnuts. Omega-3 fats have also been shown to relieve the pain of arthritis.

Unhealthy fats include saturated and trans fats. Eating too much of these unhealthy fats raises your bad cholesterol, which clogs the arteries and increases your risk of heart disease. Saturated fats are found in marbled red meats, poultry skin, coconuts, coconut oil, palm kernel oil, and whole milk products, such as milk, butter, ice cream, and cheese.

Trans fats, unlike unsaturated and saturated fats, do not exist in natural, whole foods. They are created through a chemical process called "hydrogenation," in which food manufacturers take once-healthy unsaturated fats and turn them into trans-fatty acids. Studies have shown these chemically altered fats to be potentially harmful.

Hydrogenation can add to the shelf life of a product and change a food's texture, hence its attractiveness to many food companies. To find out if your cookies, cereal, cake, peanut butter, or crackers contain trans-fatty acids, look for the words *shortening, hydrogenated oil,* or *partially hydrogenated oil* in the list of ingredients.

The 90/10 Plan strategically limits the amount of total fat in all three levels of the fourteen-day meal plans—with the majority coming from unsaturated sources (the good fat). I've intentionally left room for some saturated fat (the bad fat), which comes from your Fun Food choice. In the end, your collective fat is less than 30 percent of the day's total calories, with less than 10 percent coming from saturated sources.

Does Metabolism Really Change with Age?

Like everything else, the metabolism (the time it takes for your body to burn calories) gets slower with age. In fact your energy needs drop about 2 percent with each passing decade of adulthood. Also, when you get older you tend to lose lean body mass (muscle), which causes an even greater decrease in your metabolic rate. A diet that worked wonders for you at age eighteen probably wouldn't have the same efficiency twenty years later.

No matter what your age, however, you can still lose weight or maintain your ideal weight by being careful about what you eat and making sure that you treat your body to lots of exercise. They say that exercise keeps you younger, and it's absolutely true. The more you exercise, the more lean body mass you maintain, which offsets your natural biological decline in metabolism.

Do I Need to Take a Multivitamin/Mineral Supplement?

Some people in the nutrition field advise against taking a daily multivitamin/mineral supplement. Their logic is simply that it's better to eat your nutrients, because the body prefers nutrients in food form, not in a tablet.

Although this is true, your body requires thirteen vitamins and at least twenty-two minerals in order to carry out all its amazing, intricate, and countless jobs. Most of us, even if our diets are grounded in healthful foods, usually fall short of at least a few important nutrients each day. Plus, a calorie-restrictive diet makes getting everything you need an even greater challenge.

To support health and immunity, I advise both men and women to take a regular one-a-day multivitamin/mineral that supplies 100 percent of the recommended dietary allowances, simply as backup. It can't do anything but good. Try to take your supplements with food, and at a regular time each day, so that you make it a habit.

Will I Need a Calcium Supplement on the 90/10 Plan?

Whether you're on the 90/10 Weight-Loss Plan or not, getting adequate calcium is a must for women because women are at a greater risk for osteoporosis, the demineralization and weakening of bones.

Daily calcium requirements are high: 1,000 milligrams for women nineteen to fifty years of age, 1,200 milligrams for women over fifty who are on hormone replacement therapy, and 1,500 milligrams for women over fifty who are not. This requires three to five servings of a calcium-rich food source every single day, which can be extremely difficult on a weight-loss regimen. Make sure you're getting enough with calcium supplements in the form of calcium carbonate or calcium citrate—and split up the dose into 500 to 600 milligrams twice a day to maximize the absorption rate. Taking an entire 1,000 milligrams at once will not allow your body to adequately absorb all the calcium.

Further, if you are over fifty years of age, or have some degree of osteoporosis already, pick up a calcium supplement with vitamin D, which will enhance the absorption of calcium into the bone. Note that vitamin D is a fat-soluble vitamin, which means that it can become toxic when taken in large amounts.

Check all of your supplements, which on the 90/10 Plan includes a multivitamin/mineral and calcium pills. Make sure that your total for vitamin D does not exceed 800 IUs per day.

Will Eating Slowly Enhance My Ability to Lose Weight?

Eating slower can help you to eat less food. People who gobble down their food in record time tend to eat more than their bodies need. If you eat fast, you may not realize that your appetite has been satisfied until after you have gone overboard. Inhaling your meal also sets you up for impaired digestion and an upset stomach.

No matter how fast you eat today, you can work to slow down your pace. How? It's very simple: enjoy your food. You might laugh at such a suggestion, because most speedy eaters believe that they love meal times, snack times, party times, any times. Yet eating fast is often linked to guilty emotions about eating or being overly hungry, which is often due to waiting too long between meals. Speedy eaters often feel anxious about the whole food/weight-loss issue. They feel nervous, and so they eat fast.

Take the time to smell your food before you eat it, and experience how good it feels to smell tasty food when you're hungry. Then take a bite and concentrate on how the texture of the food feels in your mouth. Place your fork down after every two or three bites, and wait at least thirty to sixty seconds before lifting it up again for another bite. Try to remain this conscious throughout your meal. Forget reading, or working, or watching television while you're eating. Your books, paperwork, and television will all be waiting for you after your meal is finished.

If you are dining with a friend, enjoy conversation between bites. Concentrate on how great food tastes when you're hungry, and then notice how the pleasure of eating somewhat diminishes as you continue your meal and become less hungry. Stick with it—repetition creates newer, healthier habits.

Does Varying Your Food Make a Difference in Weight Loss?

It may. Varying your food can keep you from getting bored, which might keep you from eventually straying and overeating. Also, whether you are aiming to lose weight or to maintain your goal weight, varying your food allows you to nourish your body with a wide range of foods that will provide the full spectrum of nutritional benefits. That is why I encourage you to try as many of the menu ideas as you can on the 90/10 Plan.

Certainly, though, the plan was developed so that if you choose to have the same breakfast on most days, or the same lunch or the same dinner, you'll still lose weight.

However, sampling many menu ideas within the plan will supply your body with a wide variety of vitamins, minerals, and phytochemicals. After you have followed the plan for a week, you might want to look for the meals that you've been missing and give a few of them a try. This will keep your interest in the plan running smoothly while also treating your body to a broader range of nutrients.

*   *   *

Stephanie: How She Dropped Her Baby (Pregnancy) Fat

Stephanie was thirty-two and a new, first-time mom when she came to see me. She had just given birth to a baby boy, Evan Scott, who was then seven months old. Thanks to generous portions of candy, chips, and cookies, Stephanie had packed on an extra fifty pounds during pregnancy. She also nursed Evan for the first three months following his birth, which increased her appetite, making it difficult for her to curb her eating.

After the delivery, Stephanie had managed to drop twenty of those pounds by herself, which still left her with thirty pounds of added girth. During her first visit, at 5'6" she weighed in at approximately 160 pounds. Because Stephanie has a petite frame and was used to weighing 130 before being pregnant, those extra thirty-plus pounds really made a difference.

Extra pounds were something new to the once slim New Yorker, and not being able to just effortlessly drop the weight was very frustrating for Stephanie. She told me that she could fit into hardly any of her pre-pregnancy clothes so she was still wearing her maternity clothes, along with two new dresses in her "newly expanded" size, which made her feel even more miserable.

"I tried to diet here and there, and I was doing abdominal exercises 'til the cows came home, but nothing was working," remembers Stephanie. "It was extremely depressing and I was beginning to feel hopeless. Evan is the first grandson for both my parents and my husband's, so you can imagine the fuss that was made. I had two new grandmothers constantly popping over with edible goodies and cooking up feasts that were very hard to resist."

After Stephanie recorded her food for several days, it was very clear that she had a terrific metabolism. She was averaging 2,500 calories a day and she was maintaining, not gaining. Plus, since she was doing abdominal exercises yet skimping on the cardio, I knew that the 1,600-calorie 90/10 Plan, along with an extra aerobic boost, would give Stephanie quick, dramatic results.

"I really liked the 90/10 Weight-Loss Plan, as sweets are so much a part of my day that it would be hard to give them up completely," Stephanie explains. "I'm a freelance writer and I work at my computer at home. During that mid-afternoon slump I always go for the treats. I couldn't believe a diet could actually accommodate that bad food habit of mine."

The 90/10 Plan would allow Stephanie to reach for one Fun Food during her usual snack time, yet it would require her to practice portion control.

"Of course, I had to substantially cut down on the amount of candy and chips I would eat during one afternoon," Stephanie says. "But I just ate slower and savored every bite. When I was thirty pounds overweight and still going for the Milano cookies, I would feel guilty for indulging and I think that made me eat faster. Now there's no anxiety, no guilt. I know I can bask in chocolate and still maintain my ideal weight, so I'm able to relax and enjoy my Fun Food."

Together we plotted enough meals and snacks in her day so that she was never going too long without food and she was always satiated. Because doing aerobic exercise would greatly help our efforts, Stephanie joined a gym in Manhattan that had a "baby drop-off." Three days a week she took an hour-long aerobics class, usually doing low-impact, Spinning, and hip-hop to keep it varied and fun. She also joined a once-a-week strollercize group where she exercised with eight other new moms, with their small children in strollers. After fourteen days of following the 90/10 Plan and sticking to her four-days-a-week exercise routine, Stephanie weighed in seven pounds lighter.

"I used to work out before I had Evan, but after he was born I used him as an excuse not to exercise," says Stephanie. "Joy made me see that when there's a will there's a way, and nobody really has a valid excuse for not fitting in exercise. My gym has a big glass window next to the aerobics room that looks into the daycare facility, so I can watch Evan while I work out. And I love my strollercize group, as most of the women are in the same boat as I am, with regard to losing the extra pregnancy weight!"

Three-and-a-half months after she started the 90/10 Plan, Stephanie was back in her old clothing, weighing in at 132 pounds.

"I have a journal that I kept during the 90/10 Plan and I am going to keep it," says Stephanie. "I plan on using it as a reference after I have my second baby, or if I ever feel myself slipping back into any old habits."

CHAPTER THREE

Measure Your 90/10 Success: Size, Body Fat, Goal Weight, and More!

Goals are important. They can boost motivation. When you're feeling unfocused, your goals can inspire you, giving you the extra discipline necessary to stick with it. Since they are crucial to your success, goals should be set with realistic expectations. Unreasonable goals don't work.

The 90/10 Weight-Loss Plan aims to help you achieve your best. Your goal is to create a body that looks fabulous and feels healthy, light, and strong.

The most common goal-setting mistake involves your perceived target weight. Although you may have in mind a specific weight at which you think you will have achieved your best look and feel, you will do yourself a disservice if you focus on that number beyond all else. Since muscle weighs significantly more than body fat, if you are muscular it is possible to weigh more than someone of the same height as you and yet be leaner, stronger, and healthier.

When it comes to goals, you need something tangible by which to measure your success. One or all of the following methods will help you to do so—while you keep in mind that improving how you look and feel are your most important goals. Keeping track of your progress should just fuel your motivation!

FEEL GREAT!

The most important goal of the 90/10 Plan is to improve the way you feel: when you feel better physically, you will also feel more confident. Overeating takes its toll on your digestive system and energy level. Eating less and losing weight will give you more vigor and increased confidence, and you will also feel more comfortable moving, walking, working, and playing.

Take the time to notice how you feel: energetic, in control, and satisfied—not deprived. Keeping your "feel great" goal in mind is extremely important, as it will remind you that following the 90/10 Weight-Loss Plan is something you're doing for you and nobody else. Remember that the number-one goal of the 90/10 Plan is to help you feel as good as you possibly can, so that you can reap more pleasure from life.

SMILE—YOU'RE ON CAMERA!

How you look affects how you feel. Noticing how your body changes during the course of the 90/10 Plan is a huge incentive to keep going.

To record your "visual progress," have a supportive friend or family member take a photograph of you. Then, after you have followed the 90/10 Plan for at least two weeks and have exercised regularly, have another photo taken. Compare the two photos. Look for subtle changes. Maybe your waist will look a little thinner or your thighs will appear a bit firmer.

The changes that you are able to detect will empower you. You will have actual proof that your body is responding to all of your hard work. Remember: You are in control of the way your body will look.

BODY FAT VERSUS LEAN BODY MASS: YOUR WEIGHT DISTRIBUTION

How is it that two people of the same height and weight can sometimes look drastically different?

One may be small and lean, with a flat stomach and muscular, toned arms and legs, while the other may be larger, with a protruding stomach and flabby limbs—yet their weights register the same on a scale. How can that be?

It's because the smaller, leaner individual has more muscle than body fat. Muscle looks compact and firm. Fat weighs less but it takes up more space than muscle and, to state the obvious, fat makes you look fatter.

Your weight reflects the sum total of *all* your body parts—it doesn't measure your body composition, which is the amount of body fat and muscle mass you're carrying. In fact some people may register a bit high on the weight chart but actually have very little body fat, indicating that the weight is coming from firm, beautiful muscle—*not* flabby blubber.

To keep track of your muscle gains, record how many push-ups you can do. Place your hands flat on the floor, directly under your shoulders, then raise yourself up on your toes. Make sure that your body forms a straight line from your head to your heels (those who lack strength often allow their hips to raise higher than their shoulders). Slowly bend your elbows, lowering your chest to the floor. When your entire body is approximately one inch from the floor, hold the position, then slowly raise.

After regularly working on your upper body strength, you will be able to do more push-ups. An increase in strength registers an increase in muscle mass—an important goal of the 90/10 Plan. You can also record your strength gains in other exercises, such as lunges, squats, and abdominal crunches.

RUNNING THE NUMBERS

For courageous individuals who desire a more scientific approach to monitoring their fat-to-muscle ratio, here are some ways to test yourself:

Skin-Fold Calipers: Calipers resemble a handgun with salad tongs. The person who tests your body fat will grab the fat from your upper arms, lower stomach, and thighs, so that the fat is pulled away from your muscle and bone (sounds painful—it's not). The calipers will register a number from your legs, stomach, and arms. The tester will then plug these numbers into a formula to calibrate your overall body-fat percentage.

However, because some testers pinch some muscle along with fat, *or* will not pinch enough fat, results vary according to each individual tester. Therefore, if you choose the calipers method, try to return to the same tester to record your progress. Don't get "pinched" after working out, though. Exercise causes skin to swell slightly, which will register as a higher percentage of body fat than you actually are carrying.

Underwater Weighing: Getting "dunked" is the most accurate method of body-fat testing. First you sit on a scale that is situated in a small pool of warm water. As you are being lowered under the water, you blow the air out of your lungs.

When you are completely submerged (for about five seconds) your underwater weight registers on a digital scale. Then a formula determines your body fat, based on the difference between your above-water and underwater weight.

Bio-Electrical Impedance: Getting "zapped" requires that you lie on your back with one electrode attached to your hand and another to your foot.

A signal is then sent from one electrode to the other. The faster the signal travels, the more muscle you have. On the other hand, the slower the signal moves, the more fat you have, as fat impedes, or blocks, the signal.

After you've determined your body-fat percentage, compare your results with the normative ranges in the charts on the following page.

Percent Body Fat for Women

Age	Good	Excellent
20–29	20.6–22.7	17.1–19.8
30–39	21.6–24.0	18.0–20.8
40–49	24.9–27.3	21.3–24.9
50–59	28.5–30.8	25.0–27.4
60+	29.3–31.8	25.1–28.5

Percent Body Fat for Men

Age	Good	Excellent
20–29	14.1–16.8	9.4–12.9
30–39	17.5–19.7	13.9–16.6
40–49	19.6–21.8	16.3–18.8
50–59	21.3–23.4	17.9–20.6
60+	22.0–24.3	18.4–21.1

YOU GOT SMALLER! WHAT ARE YOUR CLOTHING SIZE AND MEASUREMENTS?

Before starting the 90/10 Weight-Loss Plan, record your clothing size and how well it fits. Get out your tape measure and record the measurements of your upper arms, waist, hips, and upper thighs.

Then notice when your pants start to fit you a bit looser. After you have followed the 90/10 Plan for at least two weeks, get out your tape measure again and see if you have lost a quarter-inch, or even a half-inch, from anywhere.

From which areas you lose will depend upon your genetics. Some people will lose girth from their waist first, while others will lose from their thighs. You can't control where you'll lose weight first. As I said, it's all in your genes.

YOUR GOAL-WEIGHT RANGE

The most popular method of determining success is the bathroom scale. Sure, weighing yourself is easy, convenient, and totally private, but be careful not to put all your eggs in this basket. Never judge your progress solely by your weight. Weights fluctuate due to such things as water retention, muscle gains, and, for women, the menstrual cycle.

Since your priority is to look and feel your absolute best, you cannot know your goal weight until after you have achieved your best look and feel. Because the scale does offer a quick way to gauge yourself, however, you may give yourself a carefully selected goal-weight range, based on the chart that follows, keeping in mind that this range is always subject to change.

Do not allow the normal water fluctuations in weight to discourage you. If you have stuck to the plan and have exercised regularly, a small gain is nothing to sweat. You might find yourself looking fit and firm, and being able to fit into your old jeans, yet weighing more than you thought you would.

To figure out your realistic goal-weight range, first determine your frame size with this quick-and-easy test (you will need a tape measure or calipers; you should also be wearing a short-sleeved or sleeveless top):

Extend your right arm in front of your body and bend it at a 90-degree angle, so that your upper arm is parallel to the floor and your fingers are pointing up in the air. With your left hand, find the right elbow's two protruding bones. That should represent the broadest points of your right elbow. Then, with your tape measure or calipers, determine the distance between these two bones. Be careful not to bend or round the tape while taking these measurements, or your results will be inaccurate.

The following values are for a medium frame size—anything less is considered a small frame size, anything more is considered a large frame size.

Medium Frame Size for Women

Height (no shoes)	Elbow Breadth
4'9"–5'2"	2¹/4"–2¹/2"
5'3"–5'10"	2³/8"–2⁵/8"
5'11"	2¹/2"–2³/4"

Medium Frame Size for Men

Height (no shoes)	Elbow Breadth
5'1"–5'2"	2¹/2"–2⁷/8"
5'3"–5'6"	2⁵/8"–2⁷/8"
5'7"–5'10"	2³/4"–3"
5'11"–6'2"	2³/4"–3¹/8"
6'3"	2⁷/8"–3¹/4"

Now that you've determined your frame size with the previous exercise, you may use the following chart as a guideline for your personal weight range. Keep in mind that a height/weight chart should be used only as a guideline. You may measure as having a medium frame, but look and feel fabulous at the large frame weight. And because muscle weighs more than fat, an incredibly fit person carries dense muscle and thus possibly weighs more than the chart indicates for their given height.

Weight Ranges for Women

Height	Small Frame	Medium Frame	Large Frame
4'10"	81–86	87–93	94–99
4'11"	86–91	92–98	99–105
5'0"	90–95	96–103	104–110
5'1"	95–101	102–108	109–116
5'2"	99–106	107–114	115–121
5'3"	104–111	112–119	120–127
5'4"	108–116	117–124	125–132
5'5"	113–121	122–129	130–138
5'6"	117–125	126–134	135–143
5'7"	122–130	131–139	140–149
5'8"	126–134	135–144	145–154
5'9"	131–140	141–150	151–160
5'10"	135–144	145–155	156–165
5'11"	140–150	151–160	161–171
6'0"	144–154	155–165	166–176

Weight Ranges for Men

Height	Small Frame	Medium Frame	Large Frame
5'2"	106–114	115–122	123–130
5'3"	112–120	121–128	129–136
5'4"	117–125	126–134	135–143
5'5"	122–131	132–141	142–150
5'6"	128–137	138–147	148–156
5'7"	133–142	143–152	153–163
5'8"	139–148	149–158	159–169
5'9"	144–154	155–165	166–176
5'10"	149–160	161–171	172–183
5'11"	155–166	167–177	178–189
6'0"	160–171	172–183	184–196
6'1"	166–177	178–189	190–202
6'2"	171–183	184–196	197–209
6'3"	176–189	190–203	204–216
6'4"	182–195	196–209	210–222
6'5"	187–201	202–216	217–229
6'6"	193–207	208–222	223–235

YOUR BODY-MASS INDEX (BMI)

Body-Mass Index (BMI) has been replacing height and weight tables as an index of healthy weight. The BMI is not gender specific, so it is useful for everyone.

Following on pages 76 and 77 is a BMI table that you can use to help you determine whether your current weight poses any health-related risks.

The general rule is that a BMI of 24.9 or less is considered normal and is associated with the lowest risks of obesity-related diseases. If your BMI is between 25 and 29.9 you are considered to be overweight, which increases your risk for several health complications, including heart disease and certain cancers, such as breast and ovarian. If your BMI is 30 or higher you are considered obese, with maximum health risks.

The obesity category is actually broken into three classes. Class 1 pertains to a BMI range between 30 and 34.9. Class 2 pertains to a BMI range between 35 and 39.9. And class 3 pertains to a BMI of 40 or more. As the numbers get higher, of course, the health risks become greater.

Extra weight due to increased muscle mass has not been found to cause health complications, so if you are extremely muscular your BMI reading might not be accurate. For example, two people of the same height, same weight, same age would have exactly the same BMI, but one may be incredibly fit, lean, and dense in muscle weight while the other is not physically fit, has a high percentage of body fat, and is at a very high risk for disease.

To use the following BMI table, find your height in the top row. Move down within your height column until you reach your approximate current weight (pounds have been rounded off). The number at the far right of that row is your BMI.

Body-Mass Index (BMI) Table from 4'10" through 5'6"

				HEIGHT					BMI
4'10"	4'11"	5'0"	5'1"	5'2"	5'3"	5'4"	5'5"	5'6"	
91	94	97	100	104	107	110	114	118	19
96	99	102	106	109	113	116	120	124	20
100	104	107	111	115	118	122	126	130	21
105	109	112	116	120	124	128	132	136	22
110	114	118	122	126	130	134	138	142	23
115	119	123	127	131	135	140	144	148	24
119	124	128	132	136	141	145	150	155	25
124	128	133	137	142	146	151	156	161	26
129	133	138	143	147	152	157	162	167	27
134	138	143	148	153	158	163	168	173	28
138	143	148	153	158	163	169	174	179	29
143	148	153	158	164	169	174	180	186	30
148	153	158	164	169	175	180	186	192	31
153	158	163	169	175	180	186	192	198	32
158	163	168	174	180	186	192	198	204	33
162	168	174	180	186	191	197	204	210	34
167	173	179	185	191	197	204	210	216	35
172	178	184	190	196	203	209	216	223	36
177	183	189	195	202	208	215	222	229	37
181	188	194	201	207	214	221	228	235	38
186	193	199	206	213	220	227	234	241	39
191	198	204	211	218	225	232	240	247	40
196	203	209	217	224	231	238	246	253	41
201	208	215	222	229	237	244	252	260	42
205	212	220	227	235	242	250	258	266	43
210	217	225	232	240	248	256	264	272	44
215	222	230	238	246	254	262	270	278	45
220	227	235	243	251	259	267	276	284	46
224	232	240	248	256	265	273	282	291	47
229	237	245	254	262	270	279	288	297	48
234	242	250	259	267	278	285	294	303	49
239	247	255	264	273	282	291	300	309	50
244	252	261	269	278	287	296	306	315	51
248	257	266	275	284	293	302	312	322	52
253	262	271	280	289	299	308	318	328	53
258	267	276	285	295	304	314	324	334	54

WEIGHT

Body-Mass Index (BMI) Table from 5'7" through 6'3"

| | | | | HEIGHT | | | | | BMI |
5'7"	5'8"	5'9"	5'10"	5'11"	6'0"	6'1"	6'2"	6'3"	
121	125	128	132	136	140	144	148	152	**19**
127	131	135	139	143	147	151	155	160	**20**
134	138	142	146	150	154	159	163	168	**21**
140	144	149	153	157	162	166	171	176	**22**
146	151	155	160	165	169	174	179	184	**23**
153	158	162	167	172	177	182	186	192	**24**
159	165	169	174	179	184	189	194	200	**25**
166	171	176	181	186	191	197	202	208	**26**
172	177	182	188	193	199	204	210	216	**27**
178	184	189	195	200	206	212	218	224	**28**
185	190	196	202	208	213	219	225	232	**29**
191	197	203	209	215	221	227	233	240	**30**
198	203	209	216	222	228	235	241	248	**31**
204	210	216	222	229	235	242	249	256	**32**
211	216	223	229	236	242	250	256	264	**33**
217	223	230	236	243	250	257	264	272	**34**
223	230	236	243	250	258	265	272	279	**35**
230	236	243	250	257	265	272	280	287	**36**
236	243	250	257	265	272	280	287	295	**37**
242	249	257	264	272	279	288	295	303	**38**
249	256	263	271	279	287	295	303	311	**39**
255	262	270	278	286	294	302	311	319	**40**
261	269	277	285	293	302	310	319	327	**41**
268	276	284	292	301	309	318	326	335	**42**
274	282	291	299	308	316	325	334	343	**43**
280	289	297	306	315	324	333	342	351	**44**
287	295	304	313	322	331	340	350	359	**45**
293	302	311	320	329	338	348	358	367	**46**
299	308	318	327	338	346	355	365	375	**47**
306	315	324	334	343	353	363	373	383	**48**
312	322	331	341	351	361	371	381	391	**49**
319	328	338	348	358	368	378	389	399	**50**
325	335	345	355	365	375	386	396	407	**51**
331	341	351	362	372	383	393	404	415	**52**
338	348	358	369	379	390	401	412	423	**53**
344	354	365	376	386	397	408	420	431	**54**

WEIGHT

Source: National Heart, Lung, and Blood Institute, P.O. Box 30105, Bethesda, MD 20824-0105

WHAT FACTORS DETERMINE SUCCESS?

What You Can Control

Mind Over Matter: Like anything worth achieving in life, getting into your best possible shape requires patience, discipline, and setting realistic goals. Take the time to monitor what's going on in your head. Are you doubting your ability to adopt a regular exercise routine? Are your past failures undermining your belief in yourself?

You might want to keep a journal so that you can write down your lapses in confidence and your self-defeating thoughts. Getting these thoughts on paper can help you see them in a realistic light and will give your self-doubts less control over you. Your belief in your ability to achieve success with the 90/10 Weight-Loss Plan may vary depending on the day and your mood. Just remember that lapses in confidence are a normal part of being human.

Food Intake: It may be the most difficult part of getting in shape—learning to eat less and yet feel satisfied. It is a simple fact, however, that to lose weight you must eat fewer calories than you burn off.

Think back to a time in your life when you gained weight. Well, during that time you would have been continuously eating more calories than you were burning off. When you eat less than you burn, your body is forced to burn stored fat for fuel. This is the goal of the 90/10 Plan.

However, since the 90/10 Plan includes "nondietetic" treats, you will feel more satisfied and less deprived than with a more restrictive diet. Satisfaction combined with calorie control is the key to successful weight loss.

Exercise Level: Physical activity can significantly help you reach your goals because exercise burns calories. Exercise also increases muscle mass (your lean body mass), which will increase the rate at which your body burns calories—muscle burns more calories than fat, even at rest. And exercise will help you look sleek, toned, and fit, while boosting energy levels and mood.

Of course, I should also mention that those who exercise regularly are simultaneously decreasing their chances of developing many life-threatening illnesses, such as heart disease, diabetes, and many types of cancer. Never underestimate the empowering gifts of exercise!

Metabolism: The rate, or speed, at which your body burns calories is called your metabolism. Since muscle burns the most calories, exercising regularly and gaining muscle raises your metabolism. This allows you to eat more without gaining weight, and also allows you to lose weight more quickly than someone who is carrying less muscle and more fat.

All exercise, whether it is aerobic (like running, walking, or biking) or anaerobic (like weight-lifting), can help to increase your lean body mass (in other words, build muscle), and thus raise your metabolism.

You can lower your metabolism if you go without food for a long period of time or if you follow a diet that restricts daily calories to less than 1,000. This is because your body comes equipped with what is known as the "starvation mechanism." When your body is deprived of nourishment, the starvation mechanism kicks in and your metabolism slows down to conserve energy. Inactive people with poor muscle tone who skip meals often have a slow metabolism.

If you are guilty of any or all of the above, you can work to raise your metabolism by eating regular meals and starting an exercise program that includes aerobic activity and strength training.

What You Can't *Control*

Age: Your metabolism slows as you get older. Although you can try to fight the inevitable with muscle-building exercises and cardio workouts, the bitter truth is that you may not be able to regain the speedy metabolism of your youth.

One of my clients, a forty-two-year-old woman, showed me a photo of herself at her ideal weight and appearance. It had been taken during her high school years and she was wearing her cheerleading uniform. She was seventeen years old.

Goals must be realistic in order to work. Aiming to look as you did twenty-plus years ago can be greatly discouraging as you'll likely never reach that impossible dream. With age, not only does skin get looser but it also becomes easier to gain fat and harder to build muscle. This doesn't mean you can't look incredible and feel better than you have in years, it only means that your goal should be to look and feel as good as you can *today*—not as you did twenty years ago.

Frame Size: Genetics plays a significant role in determining your body frame. Is your build small, medium, or large? To determine your size, see the chart earlier in this chapter. After you've determined your size, you can select whether your ideal weight is toward the beginning, middle, or end of your range.

The fact that we each have different genetic makeup dictates that you must strive to achieve your *own* personal best—not anyone else's. Your personal best is as healthy, fit, strong, and lean as you can be. Once you achieve that, you shouldn't want to trade it for anyone else's best!

Shape: Genetics can also determine where you tend to carry fat. Those who are pear-shaped carry excess fat in the hip/thigh/buttocks area; apple shapes carry their extra pounds around the midsection; hour-glass figures tend to be very curvaceous and store fat evenly all over. And, of course, there are other family traits that may also have been passed down to you, including fat calves, large arms, a double chin, and so on. The good news is that every single body shape looks beautiful and sexy when it is fit and strong.

Conversely, all body shapes look less than lovely when they carry excess fat and lack muscle tone. If you are unhappy with your body, it is not your shape you should aim to change but perhaps your size and your level of fitness. Once you reach your goals on the 90/10 Plan, you should be very happy with your own unique shape!

Metabolism: You can raise your metabolism with exercise, as you have just read. Genetics, however, also play an important role in metabolism. We all know someone who is genetically blessed—he or she can eat and eat and never gain a pound. This person probably finds it difficult to *gain* weight, the poor thing.

Those of us with sluggish metabolisms have a lot more company in the world. To boost your own rate of calorie-burning, lengthen your workouts or increase their frequency. Also stick to the 90/10 Plan, and work to attain the most valuable virtue in the weight-loss process: p-a-t-i-e-n-c-e.

SMALL GOALS, ONE DAY AT A TIME

Losing weight is a gradual process. Breaking your goals into mini-goals can help the day-to-day process seem a lot more feasible.

For example, if you have your heart set on dropping two clothing sizes, first aim to feel your current size fitting a tad looser. Then, after you have achieved this, aim to fit into, or almost fit into, the next smaller clothing size. If you prefer to measure success by the scale, strive to knock off two to five pounds at a time.

Some people do very well determining their progress by the scale alone, while others become obsessed with it. Figure out what works best for you. If you find the scale to be a great motivator, you can hop on it once every morning if you choose. On the other hand, if you find that it's driving you nuts, limit your weigh-ins to once a week. Or you might want to weigh yourself only outside your home, such as at the gym or your doctor's office.

If you choose to track your body fat with the caliper, make sure you return to the same trainer for another test approximately once a month. Body measurements can be taken every two weeks or so, keeping in mind that premenopausal females often swell larger, due to water retention, approximately one week before menstruation begins.

And, of course, there are no limits to how many times you can check in with yourself to determine how you're feeling! Make the connection between healthy living and feeling great as often as you can!

*   *   *

Irene and Sheldon: Now That's Teamwork!

Irene, sixty-two, and her husband, Sheldon, sixty-three, had retired to Boca Raton, Florida, from their home in New Jersey. They had been there only five short months when they realized they'd each put on about fifteen pounds, in addition to the ten or so pounds each was overweight at the time of their retirement.

"I guess it was the laid-back lifestyle and all the great restaurants all around us," says Irene. "Part of the reason that Sheldon and I chose Florida was because we loved playing tennis and golf, but the extra weight was making us feel sluggish and unenthusiastic about our favorite sports."

Eager to tackle the weight gain before it really got out of hand, Irene and Sheldon decided, together, that they would investigate the latest nutritional research, check out the popular diets, and map out a course of action.

"We weren't impressed with most of the diets, mainly because they were unrealistic for the way we like to eat," remembers Sheldon. "We were looking for something easy and normal, something that would let us enjoy our time with our grandchildren when they came to visit and we took them out for lunch."

After nixing popular diet plans, Irene called me in New York. We had first met when she came into Manhattan with her daughter, Victoria, who had been diagnosed with gestational diabetes while pregnant. At that time, we worked out a meal plan for Victoria, her pregnancy went smoothly, and soon beautiful Jennifer was born.

This time, however, Irene was calling me about herself and Sheldon. After talking with her about the lifestyle they had adopted since their move, it was easy to see why the couple had packed on the pounds—they were eating practically all their meals at restaurants that served larger-than-life portions, and they were finishing most of those portions.

The town they had moved to had so many restaurants that they were all in fierce competition with each other. Irene told me there was a breakfast joint that offered quite a deal. For $1.50, she would get a toasted bagel with butter, two scrambled eggs, hash browns, a raisin muffin, a glass of orange juice, and coffee. That computed to 1,200 calories, which is what some women who are trying to lose weight require for an entire day.

As well, Irene and Sheldon were usually eating lunches that were arranged by some organization or another at restaurants or at the country club. Their lunches sounded more like full-course dinners: bread, appetizers, entrées, and dessert. Believe it or not, Irene and Sheldon had gotten into the habit of following these huge lunch meals with an early-bird-special dinner! The portions were so huge for dinner that they would request doggie bags, and then end up finishing the leftovers while watching television later that evening.

I explained to Irene that the 90/10 Weight-Loss Plan would allow them to continue their current lifestyle, albeit with a few changes. While they could continue to eat most of their meals out, the 90/10 Plan educated them on proper serving sizes while allowing them *one* dessert a day or simply a larger portion of an entrée they loved.

Irene and Sheldon never exercised after dinner, and their nightly meals out were going straight to the fat-storage centers on their stomachs and thighs. Since Irene had always enjoyed cooking when she lived in New Jersey, they agreed to eat at home four nights during the week and found that they loved each one of the 90/10 Plan dinners. Irene also experimented with some of the additional 90/10 recipes. Together we made a list of rules that they would follow:

- Split entrées in restaurants.
- Order salads with the dressing on the side.
- Skip the bread basket completely.
- Order à la carte versus an entire dinner with "the works."
- No more doggie bags.
- Choose breakfasts such as cereal with skim milk, or scrambled egg whites and toast, or yogurt and fresh fruit. Avoid all breakfast bargains that pack in too much food and calories.
- Pay more and eat less!
- Walk each morning, prior to breakfast.
- Keep track of all food by using the 90/10 Food Log for the first few weeks.
- Plan weekly weigh-ins together—to stay honest and focused.
- Plan meals and snacks the night before.
- Cook dinner at home four nights per week.
- No more golf carts.

Because Irene was postmenopausal and felt that her metabolism had taken a dip in recent years, she followed the 1,200-calorie plan. Sheldon followed the 1,600-calorie plan, which is pretty much identical to Irene's but with bigger portions and a few additional foods here and there.

Together they made a great team. They motivated each other. When one of them wanted to slack off, the other would coach and inspire. Weekly weigh-ins became a ritual for the newly health-conscious couple. After each weigh-in, they would celebrate with a power walk and a healthy breakfast at a cafe that accommodated their low-fat requests.

After fourteen days on the 90/10 Weight-Loss Plan, Irene had lost three pounds and Sheldon had lost eight. They both felt slimmer, lighter, and healthier. Three-and-a-half months later, they were down a total of thirty-three pounds. This was about the same time they noticed that their tennis game improved dramatically. They once again became a doubles team to be reckoned with.

One year later, Irene has maintained her weight of 142 pounds, while Sheldon stays around 191. The best part is that they have encouraged a lot of their friends to join the program. They also recruited an exercise instructor to organize planned activities at their clubhouse. The instructor provides water aerobics twice a week, yoga three times a week, and a dance class once a week.

"We are eating less than when we first moved to Florida, but we don't really feel like we're on a diet, thank goodness," says Irene. "We pay close attention to eating smaller portions and try to walk as much as we can. And we both feel a hundred times better than when we were dragging around all that extra poundage!"

CHAPTER FOUR

Choosing the Right Plan for You

The 90/10 Weight-Loss Plan offers three different options: the 1,200-calorie plan, the 1,400-calorie plan, and the 1,600-calorie plan. Which one is right for you? The guidelines that follow will offer you a good idea of which route to choose. Keep in mind, however, that these are only general guidelines. You may fall into one category on paper, but in reality find yourself doing much better on a plan that offers less or more food.

For example, you may be someone over fifty years of age, with a sluggish metabolism and a sedentary job, who is not willing to exercise more than twice a week. So immediately you opt for the most stringent weight-loss formula, which provides you with 1,200 calories a day. But if that makes you feel too deprived or too hungry, or if you'd just like to be able to enjoy a bit more food, try the 1,400- or 1,600-calorie plan and see what happens. You may find that your unwanted weight falls off without the severity of the most restrictive plan.

On the other hand, you may categorize yourself as a candidate for the 1,600-calorie plan, but after following the plan for one week you feel unsatisfied with your weight-loss progress. In this instance you should switch to the 1,400-calorie plan and/or increase your exercise.

The 90/10 Plan is about changing the way you perceive food and dieting. It's a plan that will prove you can eat all types of food in moderation and lose weight forever. Understand that losing weight is not a race, and slow and steady is ultimately better than quick and drastic. Consistency, not speed, will make your efforts permanent and life-changing. Therefore, pick a plan that is realistic and will enable you to stick with it.

All of the plans include similar menus for breakfast, lunch, and dinner—which can certainly simplify meal preparation if there are other people in your life who are also following the 90/10 Plan. It's the subtle differences in the serving sizes of the foods that determine the calories you take in each day. That is why portion-control is so critical on each of the three food plans, no matter which plan you decide to follow.

If you're losing weight but are feeling too hungry on the 1,200-calorie plan, switch to the 1,400. Then, if you are following the 1,400 and still require more food, switch to the 1,600. You may lose a bit slower, but remember that the 90/10 Plan is about *permanent* weight loss. Also keep in mind that following a lower plan which deprives your body and mind will leave you feeling irritable and hungry—the perfect recipe for a quick weight loss followed by an even quicker weight gain, due to "rebound eating."

1,200-CALORIE PLAN

The least amount of calories recommended for good health is 1,200 per day. Even so, most people need to eat more, even on a calorie-controlled weight-loss plan.

And if you are male there is no reason to ever consider eating so little, even on a short-term basis. Men genetically possess more lean body mass than women (most women) and, therefore, benefit from faster metabolisms.

The 1,200-calorie plan is really for women who meet the criteria outlined below—and even those women may find that they need more food. (If so, they should switch to the 1,400-calorie plan immediately.)

However—and *very* important—even if you perfectly match all the criteria outlined, yet have a history of dieting, compulsive overeating, and/or a binge-eating disorder, do *not* follow the 1,200-calorie plan. Start with the 1,400-calorie plan (or 1,600-calorie plan), no matter how many pounds you have to lose, how slow your metabolism is, or how sedentary you are. Although the weight may come off slower, you do not want to risk feeling deprived and slipping off and bingeing, thus reverting to old habits.

Exercise Level: Because exercise burns calories, those who exercise regularly need more calories. If you do *not* exercise, or if you exercise two hours or less per week and your job is not very physically demanding, then you are not burning any extra calories and might want to consider the 1,200-calorie plan. If you exercise for more than two hours per week, you probably need to be eating more in order to sustain energy for your activities.

Age Factor: Postmenopausal women often experience a dip in their metabolic rate and find that they gain weight easily and have a hard time losing it. If you are over fifty, you might consider the 1,200-calorie plan, and more so if you are also sedentary and lack the muscle that burns extra calories.

Sluggish Metabolism: If you suspect that your metabolism is very slow, you also might consider the 1,200-calorie plan. You can judge your metabolism by how your diet is today. If you eat very little and still cannot lose weight, then the 1,200-calorie plan is probably for you. Or, if you find that most diets don't deliver on their weight-loss promise and you find it very difficult to shed pounds, then the 1,200-calorie plan is probably a wise choice. Keep in mind that exercise will also help move you closer to your goal, and building muscle will force your body to burn more calories, even at rest.

Two to Ten Pounds to Lose: Finally, for those lucky people who have only that minimal amount of weight to lose and would like to knock it off as quickly as possible, you can go ahead and follow the 1,200-calorie plan for a week or so, as long as you also follow the maintenance principles outlined in chapter 12.

If you don't meet any of these criteria, yet still wish to follow the 1,200-calorie plan because you want to see results as soon as possible in order to boost your motivation and spirits, you might try it for the first week but then switch to the 1,400-calorie plan after that—especially if you are an active individual.

1,400-CALORIE PLAN

Generally, the 1,400-calorie plan will work well for most all women—dieting history or not. Though some women with very sluggish metabolisms may require the lower 1,200-calorie plan, most women with moderately active lifestyles can lose weight effectively on the 1,400-calorie plan. Plus, the extra food will help to keep you satiated and will stabilize your blood-sugar levels throughout the day.

Contrary to women, most men will lose weight effortlessly eating *more* than 1,400 calories. Therefore, the 1,400-calorie plan is not an appropriate choice for the majority of male followers—with the exception of men who have a small stature and sedentary lifestyle.

Exercise Level: If you're a regular and moderate exerciser, working out three to five times per week, the 1,400-calorie plan may be right for you. Your workouts necessitate more food than 1,200 calories a day, and you should still lose steadily with 1,400 calories.

Your Appetite and Metabolism: The way you eat today also determines which plan you should follow. If you are used to eating a lot of food, if you are accustomed to going overboard on the weekends, or if you risk feeling deprived and uncomfortable, you should opt for 1,400 calories (if not more) per day.

Also, if you are presently eating a lot and maintaining your weight, not gaining, then chances are your metabolism is fairly active and your body will respond quickly to 1,400 calories a day.

Age and Gender: Most all women ages eighteen to fifty can easily lose weight on the 1,400-calorie plan. Women over fifty who regularly exercise three to five times per week should also have no problem losing weight on this plan.

If you are male and under 5'5", you may also choose to follow the 1,400-calorie plan, especially if you don't exercise often, have a sedentary lifestyle, and are not used to eating large amounts of food.

Two to Fifty Pounds to Lose: The 1,400-calorie plan is versatile. Whether you have a small or large amount of weight to lose, this plan will work for most everyone.

1,600-CALORIE PLAN

Gender and Height: This plan can work well for most all men—whether they exercise or not. If you are male, and 5'5" or taller, you should follow the 1,600-calorie plan. Men tend to have speedier metabolisms than women, and can therefore lose weight eating more food.

Women 5'6" and taller may also choose the 1,600-calorie plan. Taller people automatically have additional lean body mass, thus higher baseline metabolisms.

Exercise Level: Devoted exercisers who diligently work out at least five times per week should follow the 1,600-calorie plan. The extra calories coming from the 1,600-calorie plan will help to fuel and optimize your vigorous workouts.

Your Appetite: Hearty eaters may also opt for the 1,600-calorie plan. Remember, consistently following a food plan requires satisfaction and pleasure. If you love to eat (and who doesn't?), and feel that the other plans are not enough to satiate your hunger, then go for the 1,600-calorie plan. If you find that you haven't lost much weight after a week or so, you can always switch to 1,400 calories.

Thirty Pounds or More to Lose: The more weight you have to lose, the more food you can eat while you're losing it. That's because heavier people burn more calories per day and, therefore, can normally lose weight eating more food than a person weighing less. When the weight starts coming off and you get closer to your goal, however, you may need to step down to the 1,400-calorie plan.

*   *   *

Angela: The Incredible Shrinking Bride!

Angela was a yo-yo dieter before she tried the 90/10 Weight-Loss Plan, meaning that she was repeatedly losing weight on a stringent diet, only to slowly but surely gain it all back within a couple of months. She was twenty-nine when she called my office, very upset that her wedding was only four months away and she still had many pounds to lose. At that time she was 5'5" and 166 pounds.

To throw a bigger challenge than usual into the scenario, Angela explained that she was the manager of a family-owned Italian restaurant on Arthur Avenue in the East Bronx, an area known as "Little Italy in the Bronx" and famous for its delectable pasta, cheeses, breads, and meat dishes. Angela's restaurant was known within this tight-knit group of eateries for serving some of the best baked ziti and veal parmigiana in the neighborhood, and it also featured those old-fashioned dessert carts loaded with gourmet pastries and cakes.

Weight was an issue not only for Angela but also for her mom, dad, and younger brother. Angela grew up on meals of Italian bread, Caesar salad, pasta, cheese, and tomato sauce, plus ample red wine and rich desserts with cappuccino. Due to her up-and-down weight history her family's struggle with extra pounds, Angela didn't have much hope for losing the extra weight before her wedding, and she certainly wasn't optimistic about losing the extra weight for life!

"I wanted really, really badly to lose the weight for my wedding day," remembers Angela, "but I didn't want to disappoint myself, so I wouldn't allow myself to truly imagine losing it. I had been disappointed too many times in the past. But I remember explaining to Joy that my honeymoon wasn't until three months after the wedding, so if I could only keep the weight off 'til then . . . See, I certainly wasn't allowing myself to imagine losing the weight forever—that seemed like a pipe dream, given my experiences with weight loss."

After talking with Angela about her food habits, it was clear why she couldn't lose weight. She was eating way too many carbohydrates (pasta and bread) along with too-large portions in general, plus she was constantly picking and snacking at the restaurant. Her previous diets, on the other hand, were too tough to follow for the long haul. They were very restrictive and laden with long lists of forbidden foods. No one could be expected to stick to such harsh rules on a long-term basis. Yet when Angela eventually "fell off" one of these diets, she would berate herself for being weak, which would just cause her to overeat and gain the weight back and then some.

I told Angela that she would lose weight on either the 1,600-calorie plan or the 1,400. She opted for the 1,400-calorie plan in order to give herself a shot of inspiration and hope. Eating dessert on a diet was a totally new concept for Angela, so we talked for a while about all the Fun Foods she could fit into her weight-loss plan, and how she should estimate portions for both Fun Foods and meals.

"It took me a while to grasp the portion-control thing," admits Angela. "Before the 90/10 Plan, I was so used to just telling myself 'no cake!' 'no eclair!' It was a big change to go from 'no' to 'portion control.' It was almost a shock!"

We especially had to work on portion sizes of the foods Angela typically overate, namely pasta, large chicken and veal cutlets, and oversized meatballs. Also, since she did have control over what the chef was cooking, Angela asked him to make special, lower-in-fat dishes, like turkey meatballs, spinach lasagna, and vegetable stir-frys. I also gave her a list of popular low-fat salad dressings to buy. When the head chef saw Angela using a bottle of commercial dressing instead of his, however, it prompted him to create a low-fat dressing just for her.

"I'd always thought of my family's restaurant as the enemy in my weight-loss struggles, but Joy made me see that I could work with what I had, just eating lower-fat entrées and learning how to eye-ball reasonable serving sizes," says Angela. "After a couple of weeks of following the 90/10 Plan, I was saying thank goodness I have the restaurant to help me! It was like I stopped fighting food and start-ing working with it."

After fourteen days of following the 90/10 Weight-Loss Plan, Angela dropped seven pounds, which was very impressive, especially because we had barely even discussed exercise at this point. Due to the long hours at the restaurant, she had asked that we postpone the exercise habit at first. After following the 90/10 Plan for two weeks, though, Angela found that she had more energy and was ready to tackle the workout issue.

"I'm at the restaurant five days a week, so exercising for an hour during my two free days is no problem," says Angela. "But Joy encouraged me to add four days of exercise. Since I work ten- to twelve-hour days, we agreed that I would walk fifteen minutes before work and another fifteen minutes during each of two breaks, for a total of forty-five minutes. For my hour-long workouts on my off-work days, I use exercise videotapes at home."

With the extra exercise and continued weight loss, I encouraged Angela to move up to the 1,600-calorie plan. Even if this meant that she would lose weight slower, I felt that it was important, given her yo-yo dieting history. I didn't want her diet to be so drastically different from her usual nondiet eating habits. Angela agreed to follow the 1,600-calorie plan, yet would sometimes return to the 1,400 plan if she wasn't able to fit in four days of exercise during the week.

After the initial two weeks, Angela lost an average of two pounds a week. Although her stringent diets in the past had allowed her to lose weight at a faster pace, Angela said that they made her feel tired, cranky, and depressed. Because she was feeling energetic, satisfied, and relaxed on the 90/10 Plan, she was able to practice patience as the scale and her size slowly moved down.

"The guy who was tailoring my wedding gown used to tease me about my diminishing measurements," says Angela. "He used to call me 'The Incredible Shrinking Bride.' That made me feel great and I began to actually look forward to getting my waist measured, which would have been a source of great anguish before I started the 90/10 Plan."

For Angela's healthy and weight-conscious rehearsal dinner, the chef made grilled portabella mushrooms, a salad with the "secret" low-fat dressing he'd created for her, chicken cacciatore, and half-orders of pasta marinara. The best red wine was flowing, so Angela opted to have two glasses that day as her Fun Food.

Four months after starting the 90/10 Plan, Angela got married weighing 132 pounds—a total of thirty-four pounds less than when she walked into my office just four months earlier. She looked drop-dead gorgeous and, more important, felt rested, beautiful, and confident.

"I had never lost weight on a diet before and felt that the weight loss would be absolutely permanent," says Angela. "But I felt so satisfied on the 90/10 Plan that I knew it was forever. I think that easy confidence and inner happiness really shone through on my wedding day. People were telling me how great I looked, and that was wonderful, but what really felt special is that I felt great on the inside as well. I had been a hopeless, stressed-out, yo-yo dieter, and here I was, a peaceful and proud slim woman!"

Angela worked hard at the maintenance plan, weighing herself once a week and continuing her exercise habit. I gave her a five-pound range to fall into (130–135 pounds). If she went higher than 135 pounds, she would simply follow the 90/10 Plan for one week and lose it again.

"I feel like my entire attitude and relationship with food has changed 100 percent," says Angela. "I feel in control. No food is my enemy now. I know I can eat anything I want, as long as I practice good portion control. In fact, I now know that trying to completely resist my favorite foods, like garlic bread and red wine and canolies, will always backfire. It's much better to eat a little and satisfy a craving than resist the food completely only to overeat in another couple of days."

Angela left for her honeymoon solidly within her goal-weight range. When she returned she was only four pounds heavier, which she lost in two weeks of following the 90/10 Plan again.

"Now my little brother is on the 90/10 Plan and he's losing weight quicker than I did!" says Angela. "Watching me lose the weight, and still eat chocolate, really inspired him to go for it!"

Still eating chocolate, and still within her goal-weight range, Angela says she has no doubts that her 90/10 body is here to stay.

PART TWO

The Meal Plans, Recipes, and Fun Foods

What You Should Know Before Beginning the 90/10 Weight-Loss Plan

The following will help you to better understand some of the specifics of your 90/10 Plan. You can always refer back to this list whenever you are uncertain about particulars.

THE BASICS

The 90/10 Ratio: The 90/10 Weight-Loss Plan is a realistic food strategy, *not* exact math. In fact the numbers on this plan can range from 80 percent healthy and 20 percent fun to 100 percent healthy and 0 percent fun. It all depends on the specific plan you decide to follow and your Fun Food choice (or not). You'll also notice that some of the Fun Foods supply fun with nutrition, for example, nuts, cheese, ice cream. With that in mind, the title "90/10" is a good representative average. Bottom line: Simply enjoy eating a lot of healthy with a bit of fun!

Calorie Breakdown for Each Meal: Understanding the exact breakdown for each meal and snack can help when certain foods are not available or practical. For example, you may find yourself in a situation where you're not able to prepare a 90/10 meal and a frozen entrée from the supermarket is the best alternative. This is fine, as long as the substituted meal falls within the appropriate caloric range. You may also want to alter a few 90/10 meals to fit your personal tastes, but again, you must stay within your caloric guidelines. Keep in mind that substitutions should be kept to a minimum (no more than two per week), because these menus were designed to provide well-balanced nutrition. To replace with less healthy alternatives would be counterproductive to the 90/10 strategy.

The Calorie Breakdowns for the Three Plans

	1,200-calorie plan	1,400-calorie plan	1,600-calorie plan
Breakfast	200 calories	250 calories	250 calories
Lunch	300 calories	350 calories	400 calories
Snack	100 calories	100 calories	150 calories
Dinner	350 calories	450 calories	550 calories
Fun Food	250 calories	250 calories	250 calories

Going Overboard at a Meal: If you go off your plan completely at a meal, do *not* give up on the entire day. Simply count the excessive meal as your meal plus your Fun Food.

Severe Hunger and/or Lightheadedness: If you become extremely hungry or experience bouts of hypoglycemia (low blood sugar, which can leave you lightheaded, dizzy, and fatigued), or if you find that you simply need more food or need to eat more often than the plan provides for, incorporate an extra snack when your body requires it. First try to trim those extra calories from your dinner or lunch. But small additional snacks should not impede your weight-loss efforts. Snacks may include one serving of fruit or vegetable, a nonfat yogurt, or a slice of reduced-calorie, whole-wheat bread with a teaspoon of peanut butter or slice of low-fat cheese.

Coffee and Tea: You may drink unlimited plain coffee or tea throughout the day. If you are caffeine sensitive, however, limit your consumption. (If you are taking medication or have a preexisting medical condition, always ask your physician what caffeine allowances are suitable for you.)

Vegetables: Any vegetable listed with any dinner may be substituted with any of the following vegetables on any given night (portion size stays the same): asparagus, beets, broccoli, Brussels sprouts, cabbage, carrots, cauliflower, celery, cucumbers, eggplant, green beans, greens (collard, mustard, and turnip), kohlrabi, leeks, lettuce, mushrooms, okra, onions, pea pods, peppers (red, yellow, and green), radishes, rutabaga, spinach, tomatoes, water chestnuts, or zucchini.

Fruits: You may substitute any of the snack or dinner fruits listed on your plan with the following alternatives—but please note that these substitutions do *not* apply to breakfast or lunch. Be sure to stick with the serving size noted for each fruit: 1 medium apple, 1/2 cup unsweetened applesauce, 4 apricots, 3/4 cup blackberries, 3/4 cup blueberries, 1/4 cantaloupe (or 1 cup, cubed), 12 cherries (large, raw), 2 clementines, 2 figs, 1/2 grapefruit, 20 grapes, 1 kiwi, 1/2 mango, 1 nectarine, 1 orange, 1 peach, 1 medium pear, 2 persimmons, 1 cup pineapple, 1/2 pomegranate, 2 small plums, 2 tablespoons raisins, 1 cup raspberries, 11/2 cups strawberries (whole), 2 tangerines, 1 medium-size watermelon wedge (or 1 cup, cubed).

Milk Products: Low-fat soy milk and/or Lactaid milk may be substituted for skim milk on each of the three 90/10 food plans.

Bread: Whole-wheat bread is always preferred. However, an *occasional* substitute slice of white bread is fine. When your plan specifies reduced-calorie, whole-wheat bread, check labels carefully and buy only brands that provide no more than 40 calories per slice.

Pita Bread: When the meal plan specifies a *small* pita bread, buy brands that provide no more than 70 calories per pita. When the plan specifies a *regular*-size pita bread, buy brands that provide no more than 160 calories per pita.

Water and Non-Caloric Seltzer: Have as much as you want, whenever you'd like! You may also enjoy the non-caloric, flavored varieties of seltzer, or squeeze in your own fresh lemon.

Artificial Sweeteners: Diet beverages and other artificially sweetened foods will not impede your weight-loss efforts in any way. However, if you choose to include these items in your 90/10 Weight-Loss Plan, do so in moderation.

Seasonings: You may use unlimited amounts of the following seasonings: basil, bay leaves, celery seeds, chili powder, chives, cinnamon, cumin, curry, dill, flavoring extracts (such as almond, vanilla, and walnut), garlic powder, hot pepper sauce, lemon, lemon juice, lemon pepper, lime, lime juice, minced onion, onion powder, oregano, paprika, parsley, pepper, pimento, low-sodium soy sauce, tarragon, thyme, turmeric, and vinegar.

Chewing Gum: You may have one standard pack per day of any sugarless chewing gum you choose.

Vegetarian Adjustments: Tofu or tempeh may be substituted at any time for meat, chicken, or fish. For tofu, simply double the ounces listed in a particular meal for meat, chicken, or fish. For tempeh, ounces remain exactly the same as those listed for meat, chicken, or fish. Veggie burgers may be substituted for burgers made with beef or turkey meat.

Low-fat soy milk may be substituted for skim milk (amounts remain the same), and soy cheese or vegetable cheese may be substituted for regular low-fat/nonfat cheese (amounts remain the same).

1,200-Calorie Plan

For those of you who would like to go for the most stringent weight-loss formula, here's the 1,200-calorie plan. Each of the fourteen days has been carefully formulated to total 950 calories—leaving room for your daily Fun Food.

Each day, refer to the listings in chapter 9 to select a Fun Food of your choosing. They are all portion-controlled and provide no more than 250 calories, so that your daily totals will add up to 1,200 calories. (Note: For the sake of good health and a robust metabolism, never follow a diet that provides less than 1,200 calories a day.)

Although each meal is packed with as much calcium, fiber, vitamins, and minerals as possible, the caloric restrictions make taking a daily multivitamin/mineral supplement a good idea. Women may also consider a separate calcium supplement (see chapter 2).

Because each breakfast contains the same number of calories, if you're partial to a particular breakfast, feel free to enjoy it more than once a week. You may also substitute any of the lunches for lunches, snacks for snacks, and dinners for dinners. Be aware, however, that variety also provides your body with a variety of nutrients. And variety is the key to staying satisfied and keeping things fresh, so don't get stuck with a limited number of meals.

You can also turn to the 90/10 Recipe Appendix on page 281, where you will find ten additional delicious dinners that can be substituted for any other dinners on any night—as long as you follow the portions and accompaniments for your particular plan.

It's true that you're free to enjoy one Fun Food every single day at whatever time you choose, but you may not always be in the mood. The 90/10 Plan takes this into consideration. At the bottom of each day's menu, you'll notice a box that instructs you on healthier alternatives to add into your day if you'd rather skip the Fun Food.

Remember to drink plenty of water (or non-caloric seltzer), and pay close attention to the proper servings and amounts for all your meals. If you find that you are too hungry on this plan or you are losing weight too rapidly, switch to the 1,400-calorie plan.

DAY 1
1 , 2 0 0   C A L O R I E S

Enjoy one Fun Food at the time of day of your choosing.

Breakfast

1 serving oatmeal, prepared with water*
2 level tablespoons raisins, or 1/2 banana, or 3/4 cup berries or melon
Coffee or tea (skim milk optional)

> *Use 1 packet dry, instant oatmeal, any flavor, that is *less* than 150 calories per serving, or use 1/2 cup dry, traditional oatmeal, with cinnamon to taste.

Lunch

Open-faced tuna melt*
Water or seltzer

> *Spread 3 ounces water-packed tuna (mixed with 1 level tablespoon low-fat mayonnaise) over 2 slices toasted, reduced-calorie, whole-wheat bread. Top each half with sliced tomato, onion, and 1 slice low-fat cheese. Bake or toast until cheese melts.
>
> You may choose to skip the cheese and have an orange instead.

Snack

1 apple or pear (or 1 peach, 1/2 mango, or 1 cup fresh pineapple)

Dinner

Chicken stir-fry*

Water or seltzer

> *Stir-fry 5 ounces boneless/skinless chicken breast (cut into strips) in 2 teaspoons vegetable oil until almost cooked. Add 1½ cups mixed vegetables (snow peas, mushrooms, broccoli) and low-sodium soy sauce. Stir-fry until chicken is thoroughly cooked.

If you prefer to skip the Fun Food today, you can add 1 cup of brown rice or couscous to your dinner.

DAY 2
1,200 CALORIES

Enjoy one Fun Food at the time of day of your choosing.

Breakfast

2 slices toasted, reduced-calorie, whole-wheat bread,
    with 1 level tablespoon peanut butter
Coffee or tea (skim milk optional)

Lunch

Large tossed salad*
1/2 regular-size (or 1 small) whole-wheat pita bread
Water or seltzer

> *Combine unlimited raw lettuce, cucumbers, mushrooms, carrots, tomatoes, onions, and peppers, topped with 4 ounces grilled chicken breast or shrimp (or 2 hard-boiled eggs), with 1 tablespoon regular *or* 2 tablespoons low-fat or nonfat dressing (or 1 teaspoon olive oil and unlimited lemon or vinegar).

Snack

Frozen fruit-pop of your choice (100 calories or less)

Dinner

3-ounce turkey burger (or frozen veggie burger)*

1 cup steamed green beans

1/2 grapefruit or 1 orange

Water or seltzer

> *Prepare burger with 1 slice low-fat or nonfat cheese melted
> on top, 2 tablespoons ketchup, and lettuce, tomato, and onion
> slices (without bun).

---

*If you prefer to skip the Fun Food for the day, enjoy another
tablespoon of peanut butter with your breakfast, plus the
other half of the pita bread with your lunch, and an apple at
any point in your day.*

DAY 3
1,200 CALORIES

Enjoy one Fun Food at the time of day of your choosing.

Breakfast

Toast Hawaiian-style*

Coffee or tea with skim milk

> *Combine 1/3 cup low-fat ricotta cheese (or 1/2 cup 1% low-fat cottage cheese) with 1/4 cup crushed pineapple (packed in its own juice), drained, plus a dash of nutmeg. Spread over 2 slices toasted, reduced-calorie, whole-wheat bread.

Lunch

Lettuce/turkey rollups*

1/2 frozen banana (or 1 peach, plum, or orange)

Water or seltzer

> *Lay out a few large romaine lettuce leaves, and layer each with 3 ounces turkey breast, 1 1/2 ounces low-fat cheese (approximately 2 slices), sliced tomato, and thinly sliced cucumber. (Optional: Add 1 tablespoon low-fat salad dressing, mayonnaise, or dijon mustard.) Roll all ingredients in the outer lettuce leaves. Makes approximately 3 rolls, equivalent to 1 serving.

Snack

Low-fat hot cocoa (1 instant packet, 50 calories or less)

1/2 cup baby carrots (approximately 8 carrots)

Dinner

Steamed Chinese food*

Baked apple (see recipe, Day 12)

Water or seltzer

> *Steamed chicken, beef, or seafood (4 ounces), with unlimited vegetables (try steamed string beans, eggplant, broccoli, pea pods, mushrooms, water chestnuts), drizzled with 1 tablespoon garlic sauce, plus unlimited soy sauce (preferably the low-sodium version).
>
> (When dining in a Chinese restaurant, or ordering takeout, request the garlic sauce on the side and use only 1 tablespoon.)

If you prefer to skip the Fun Food today, add 1/2 cup white or brown rice with dinner and have an 8-ounce glass of orange juice with breakfast (preferably calcium-fortified).

DAY 4
1,200 CALORIES

Enjoy one Fun Food at the time of day of your choosing.

Breakfast

4 scrambled egg whites*

1 slice whole-wheat toast, dry (or 2 slices reduced-calorie, whole-wheat bread)

Coffee or tea (skim milk optional)

>*Scramble egg whites with 1 slice low-fat cheese and chopped tomatoes. (Use nonstick cooking spray.)

Lunch

Stuffed pita pocket*

Large pickle

Water or seltzer

>*Mix chopped lettuce, tomato, cucumbers, raw mushrooms, onion, 1/4 cup of any type of beans (or 1 ounce of shredded, low-fat cheese), with 1 tablespoon of any low-fat dressing. Stuff into a whole-wheat pita bread.

Snack

Apple or pear or 1/2 cup grapes (approximately 20 grapes)

Dinner

4-ounce lean steak or hamburger or turkey burger*
1 cup sautéed spinach, broccoli, green beans, or cauliflower**
1/4 cantaloupe or 1 1/2 cups whole strawberries
Water or seltzer

>   *Prepare preferred meat with 1 tablespoon ketchup, or barbecue or steak sauce.

>   **Sauté vegetables with 1 teaspoon olive oil, and garlic.

If you prefer to skip the Fun Food today, enjoy a medium-size baked potato (about 7 ounces) with 2 level teaspoons of a reduced-calorie, soft-tub margarine or 1 level tablespoon of reduced-fat sour cream with dinner.

DAY 5
1,200 CALORIES

Enjoy one Fun Food at the time of day of your choosing.

Breakfast

3/4 cup dry cereal*

1 cup skim or 1% milk

Coffee or tea (skim milk optional)

> *Choose a cereal variety with more than 3 grams of fiber and less than 120 calories per 3/4-cup serving, such as Bran Flakes®, Kashi to Good Friends®, Cheerios®, Total®, or All-Bran®.

Lunch

1 bowl chicken noodle, vegetable, or minestrone soup (approximately 2 cups)

5 reduced-fat Wheat Thins® crackers (or 1 slice reduced-calorie, whole-wheat bread)

Water or seltzer

Snack

1 tablespoon hummus

1 small, whole-wheat pita bread

Dinner

Egg-white omelet*

Toasted English muffin**

1/2 grapefruit or 2 clementines

Water or seltzer

*Use 5 egg whites, or 1 cup egg substitute, with spinach, mushrooms, onions, and 1 slice low-fat cheese or 1 rounded tablespoon of feta cheese. (Use nonstick cooking spray.)

**Preferably whole-wheat English muffin, and topped with 1 teaspoon margarine or butter (or 2 teaspoons of a reduced-fat spread).

If you prefer to skip the Fun Food today, enjoy a banana in your breakfast cereal, an additional 5 reduced-fat Wheat Thins® with lunch, and an apple at any point in your day.

DAY 6
1,200 CALORIES

Enjoy one Fun Food at the time of day of your choosing.

Breakfast

1 frozen whole-grain waffle*

2 tablespoons reduced-calorie light syrup

Coffee or tea (skim milk optional)

> *Any waffle brand 120 calories or less (and preferably calcium-fortified), topped with 1/2 cup sliced berries or peaches (fresh, or canned in extra-light syrup).

Lunch

3/4 cup 1% low-fat cottage cheese*

1/2 cantaloupe (or 1 cup of seasonal fresh fruit salad)

Water or seltzer

> *Mix cottage cheese with 2 tablespoons of wheat germ or low-fat granola (or other crunchy cereal). The fruit can also be mixed in with the cereal and cottage cheese.

Snack

1 granola bar or cereal bar (any bar 100 calories or less)

Dinner

Lettuce and tomato salad*

5 ounces grilled salmon**

1 cup steamed zucchini, broccoli, or spinach

1/2 grapefruit

Water or seltzer

*Drizzle lettuce and tomato with 1 teaspoon olive oil and unlimited balsamic vinegar (or 2 tablespoons low-fat dressing or 1 tablespoon of any type of regular dressing).

**Prepare salmon (or 5 ounces of any other type of fish) with 1 teaspoon olive oil and fresh lemon. Season to taste.

If you prefer to skip the Fun Food today, add to dinner a medium-size sweet potato (about 7 ounces), with 1 teaspoon margarine or butter (or 2 teaspoons of a reduced-calorie spread).

DAY 7
1,200 CALORIES

Enjoy one Fun Food at the time of day of your choosing.

Breakfast

1 cup (8-ounce container) nonfat flavored yogurt*

Coffee or tea (skim milk optional)

> *Mix yogurt with 2 tablespoons of low-fat granola cereal (or wheat germ).

Lunch

Turkey breast or lean ham sandwich*

Water or seltzer

> *Take 2 slices reduced-calorie, whole-wheat bread and layer with 3 ounces turkey breast or lean ham, 1 slice low-fat cheese, and lettuce, tomato, and mustard (optional: 1 tablespoon low-fat mayonnaise).

Snack

1 1/2 cups baby carrots (approximately 24 carrots)

Dinner

Spinach lasagna*

Sliced cucumber

Water or seltzer

> *This recipe yields 12 servings. The appropriate portion size is 1/12 of the entire lasagna. Cut into 12 servings and individually freeze remaining portions for future dinners.

2 10–12-ounce boxes frozen spinach (or broccoli), chopped

2 pounds low-fat ricotta cheese

1 whole egg plus 2 egg whites

3/4 teaspoon pepper

Garlic to taste

Basil to taste

1/2 tablespoon oregano

4 cups skim-milk mozzarella cheese, shredded

Nonstick cooking spray

1 32-ounce jar of tomato/marinara sauce (any brand less than 50 calories per 1/2-cup serving)

1 16-ounce package lasagna noodles, uncooked

1 cup water (for cooking only)

Cook and drain spinach well, then set aside. Mix together ricotta cheese, eggs, pepper, garlic, basil, oregano, and only half of the mozzarella cheese. Add in spinach and mix again thoroughly. Coat lasagna pan with nonstick spray and pre-heat oven to 350°F.

Cover the bottom of pan with tomato sauce and place down a layer of the uncooked lasagna noodles. Next, spread half of the spinach/cheese mixture evenly on top, and repeat the layers (noodles and then the remaining spinach/cheese mixture). Place one more layer of noodles on top (total of 3 noodle layers) and pour on the remaining tomato sauce. Sprinkle on the other half of the mozzarella cheese. Last, pour the water around the edge of the pan (this will cook the noodles), and cover tightly with aluminum foil. Bake for 1 hour and 15 minutes, until bubbling.

Let stand to cool for 15 minutes before slicing. Remember that one serving equals 1/12 of the entire lasagna.

If you prefer to skip the Fun Food today, you can have an extra 1/2 slice of spinach lasagna with dinner, and 1 orange or 1 peach at any point during your day.

DAY 8
1,200 CALORIES

Enjoy one Fun Food at the time of day of your choosing.

Breakfast

Chunky apple oatmeal*

Coffee or tea (skim milk optional)

> *Take 1 serving of dry oatmeal (1/2 cup) or 1 packet of instant oatmeal (regular flavor) and cook as directed. Next, peel and cut up half an apple into small bite-size pieces and mix throughout the cooked oatmeal. Sprinkle on 2 teaspoons brown sugar (optional: cinnamon) and microwave for approximately 1 minute.

Lunch

1 regular-size, whole-wheat pita bread

1/4 cup hummus

Small tossed or chopped salad*

Water or seltzer

> *Mix lettuce, onion, tomato, and peppers, and add fresh lemon. Salt and pepper to taste.

Snack

1 cup nonfat pudding, any flavor (can be bought preprepared; if made from scratch, use skim or 1% milk)

Dinner

4-ounce lean flank or sirloin steak*

Sliced tomato with plain balsamic vinegar

1 cup steamed asparagus

Water or seltzer

*Marinate steak in 3 tablespoons of teriyaki sauce (preferably low-sodium), then grill or broil.

If you prefer to skip your Fun Food today, you can enjoy an additional 2 ounces of steak with dinner (totaling 6 ounces), and an extra 1/4 cup of hummus with lunch (totaling 1/2 cup).

DAY 9
1,200 CALORIES

Enjoy one Fun Food at the time of day of your choosing.

Breakfast

1 medium (or 2 small) pancake(s)*
Coffee or tea (skim milk optional)

> *Top pancakes with 1/2 banana (sliced) or 1/2 cup of any other fresh fruit.

Lunch

Fresh tossed salad*
1 small whole-wheat pita bread, or 2 slices reduced-calorie, whole-wheat bread
Water or seltzer

> *Toss together unlimited raw vegetables (try lettuce, mushrooms, onions, cucumbers, tomatoes, carrots, broccoli). Add 1/4 cup cooked red kidney beans and 1/4 cup low-fat cottage cheese, with 1 tablespoon of any type salad dressing (or 2 tablespoons reduced-fat salad dressing, or 2 teaspoons olive oil and unlimited balsamic vinegar).

Snack

1 1/2 cups fresh, whole strawberries (or 1/2 cup sliced peaches canned in extra-light syrup)

2 rounded tablespoons reduced-calorie whipped cream (such as Light Cool Whip®)

Dinner

Shrimp and pasta primavera*

Water or seltzer

> *Sauté 1/2 cup zucchini (cut into 1-inch rounds), with 1/2 cup sliced mushrooms and 1 clove of fresh garlic, in 2 teaspoons olive oil. Add 5 ounces cooked shrimp (or 3 ounces salmon or 3 ounces chicken breast) and 1/2 cup low-sodium chicken broth to sautéed vegetables; season with basil and oregano. Pour over 1/2 cup cooked spaghetti or linguini (preferably whole-wheat).

If you prefer to skip the Fun Food today, you can add an 8-ounce glass of orange juice with your breakfast (preferably calcium-fortified), plus an additional 1/2 cup spaghetti with your dinner (totaling 1 cup).

DAY 10
1,200 CALORIES

Enjoy one Fun Food at the time of day of your choosing.

Breakfast
Fruit smoothie*
Coffee or tea (skim milk optional)

> *Blend together 1/4–1/2 cup plain or vanilla nonfat yogurt, 1/2 cup skim milk, 1/4 cup orange juice, 1/2 banana, 1/2 cup whole strawberries (or 1/4 cup sliced), and ice as desired.

Lunch
Stuffed potato*
Water or seltzer

> *Take a medium-size potato (about 7 ounces) and bake or microwave until done. Top baked potato with 1/2 cup cooked, chopped broccoli and 1 ounce shredded (or 1 1/2 small slices) low-fat or nonfat cheddar cheese. Place back in oven until cheese melts.

Snack
1 ounce of pretzels

Dinner

Flake-bake chicken*

1 cup steamed broccoli or spinach

1 orange or 1 peach

Water or seltzer

> *Preheat oven to 350°F. Take 5 ounces boneless chicken breast and dip in 1 beaten egg white. Season with garlic, pepper, minced onion, oregano, and salt to taste. Next, dip chicken breast in 1/4–1/2 cup crushed Bran Flakes® cereal and coat on both sides. Bake for approximately 30–45 minutes (ovens may vary).
>
> You may also choose to skip the egg white and instead dip chicken in teriyaki sauce, marinara sauce, or low-fat Caesar salad dressing, before covering in Bran Flakes®.

If you prefer to skip the Fun Food today, you can enjoy an extra 4–5-ounce piece of flake-bake chicken at dinner.

DAY 11
1,200 CALORIES

Enjoy one Fun Food at the time of day of your choosing.

Breakfast
Toasted whole-wheat English muffin*
Coffee or tea (skim milk optional)

   *Top English muffin with 2 slices of melted low-fat cheese.

Lunch
Mexican wrap*
Water or seltzer

   *Wrap 3 ounces of grilled chicken (cut into strips), 2–4 tablespoons salsa, fresh lettuce, and 1/2 ounce reduced-fat Monterey Jack cheese in a flour tortilla (any brand tortilla, approximately 100 calories).

Snack
Skim café latte or skim cappuccino

Dinner

Linguini with red clam sauce*

Side salad**

Water or seltzer

*Mix 1/2 cup cooked linguini (preferably whole-wheat) with 1/2 cup red clam sauce.

**Combine unlimited mixed green lettuce, 1/2 tomato cut into chunks, 1/2 cup white cannelini or garbanzo beans, and 2 tablespoons reduced-calorie salad dressing (or 1 teaspoon olive oil with unlimited lemon or vinegar).

If you prefer to skip the Fun Food today, you can enjoy an additional 1 cup pasta and 1/4 cup red clam sauce with your dinner (totaling 1 1/2 cups pasta).

DAY 12
1,200 CALORIES

Enjoy one Fun Food at the time of day of your choosing.

Breakfast

Scrambled tofu*

2 slices reduced-calorie, whole-wheat toast

Coffee or tea (skim milk optional)

> *Mash 4 ounces of firm tofu. In a separate bowl, whisk together a dash of cumin, dash of garlic powder, 1 tablespoon water, 1 1/2 teaspoons mellow-barley light miso, and fresh-ground pepper to taste. Heat tofu over medium flame and immediately add in miso mixture. Stir constantly until tofu mixture is heated through. If you choose, 2 tablespoons of ketchup can also be added before serving.

Lunch

English-muffin pizza*

Water or seltzer

> *Split and toast a whole-wheat English muffin in oven. Next, spread on marinara sauce and top with 1 ounce low-fat mozzarella cheese (part skim). Add thinly sliced tomatoes, onions, peppers, and mushrooms. Bake in oven until cheese melts.

Snack
Baked apple*

*Use Rome, McIntosh, Jonagold, or Granny Smith apple. Preheat oven to 350°F. Core apple from top to 1/2 inch from bottom. Place in shallow baking dish and sprinkle 1 teaspoon sugar and cinnamon (or nutmeg and 1 teaspoon reduced-calorie syrup) in center hole of apple. Pour minimal amount of water to coat bottom of baking dish and cover tightly with foil. Bake for 30 minutes, then uncover and bake another 5–10 minutes (until tender, but not mushy). For microwaves, cover with microwave-safe shield and check apple after 5 minutes.

Dinner
5-ounce fish filet*
1 cup spaghetti squash with 1/2 cup tomato sauce
1 cup fresh steamed green beans
Water or seltzer

*Broil fish with 1 tablespoon reduced-calorie margarine or 1 teaspoon olive oil, plus lemon juice, fresh basil, and seasoning to taste.

If you choose to skip the Fun Food today, you can enjoy a second 5-ounce fish filet with dinner, plus a 1/2 grapefruit or 1 orange (or peach or nectarine) at any point in your day.

DAY 13
1,200 CALORIES

Enjoy one Fun Food at the time of day of your choosing.

Breakfast

French raisin toast*

1/2 grapefruit or 1/4 cantaloupe

Coffee or tea (skim milk optional)

>*Coat skillet with nonfat cooking spray and heat. Mix egg substitute (or 1 egg white) with 1/2 teaspoon vanilla extract. Dip 1 slice raisin bread into mixture (coating both sides) and place in skillet. Cook until both sides are light brown. Top with 2 tablespoons (2 squirts) reduced-calorie light syrup.

Lunch

Grilled-chicken Greek salad*

1 orange or 1/2 grapefruit (or 2 cups low-calorie, diet Jell-O®)

Water or seltzer

>*Combine unlimited spinach leaves with 2 ounces grilled chicken, raw vegetables, and 1 ounce feta cheese, tossed with 1 teaspoon olive oil and unlimited plain vinegar.

Snack

1 level tablespoon peanut butter (or 2 tablespoons low-fat cream cheese) spread over 1 stalk of celery

Dinner
Vegetarian chili*

Water or seltzer

*Use any nonfat or low-fat, commercially prepared vegetarian chili, or make your own with this recipe, which yields 6 servings. The appropriate portion size is 2 cups.

1/2 cup texturized vegetable protein (TVP)

1/4 cup boiling water

1/2 tablespoon olive oil

1 large onion, diced

3 cloves garlic, minced

2 medium carrots, chopped

2 medium celery stalks, chopped

1 green bell pepper, seeded and chopped

8 ounces mushrooms, quartered

Juice of 1 lemon

1 1/2 teaspoons chili powder

1/2 teaspoon dried basil

1/2 teaspoon dried oregano

1/8 teaspoon red pepper flakes

1 1/2 teaspoons ground cumin

1 15-ounce can kidney beans

1 15-ounce can pinto beans

1 large tomato, chopped

1 28-ounce can crushed tomatoes

1/2 teaspoon Marsala wine (optional)

1 tablespoon tomato paste

2–4 tablespoons fresh chives and/or parsley (optional)

1 cup red onion, chopped

Low-fat or nonfat sour cream

Combine the TVP and boiling water in a bowl and set aside. Meanwhile, heat oil in a large stock pot, add onions, and sauté until soft (about 3 minutes). Next, add garlic, carrots, celery, bell pepper, mushrooms, lemon juice, and spices. Cook over medium heat, covered, for 5 minutes.

Stir in TVP, kidney and pinto beans, chopped tomato, and crushed tomatoes. Bring to a simmer. Cook uncovered over low heat for 15 minutes, stirring occasionally. Add Marsala wine and tomato paste, and simmer again for an additional 5 minutes. Remove pot from heat and stir in fresh herbs.

Ladle the chili into bowls and garnish with chopped red onion and 1 heaping tablespoon low-fat or nonfat sour cream. One serving equals 2 cups.

If you prefer to skip the Fun Food today, you can enjoy 1 cup (8 ounces) of orange juice with breakfast; 1 small, whole-wheat pita bread with your lunch (or 4 Melba toast crackers); and 1½ cups whole strawberries (or peach, nectarine, ½ grapefruit, or ¼ cantaloupe) at any point in your day.

DAY 14
1,200 CALORIES

Enjoy one Fun Food at the time of day of your choosing.

Breakfast

Bananas and cream*

Coffee or tea (skim milk optional)

> *Mix a sliced banana together with 2 rounded tablespoons of reduced-fat sour cream and 1–2 teaspoons sugar.

Lunch

Toasted cheese and tomato sandwich*

1 cup baby carrots (approximately 16 carrots)

Water or seltzer

> *Take 2 slices of dry, toasted, reduced-calorie, whole-wheat bread and layer with 2 ounces of any type of low-fat sliced cheese and unlimited tomato slices. Place back in oven until cheese melts.

Snack

12 reduced-fat Wheat Thins® crackers

Dinner

Chicken or steak fajitas*

Side salad**

Water or seltzer

> *Sauté 4 ounces of chicken (or lean sirloin steak) strips in fajita seasonings packet and 1 teaspoon olive oil (you may also add nonstick cooking spray). Add strips of red, green, and yellow peppers, along with sliced red onion, into the pan to sauté as the chicken cooks through. Wrap chicken (or steak), and the strips of vegetables, in 1 small flour tortilla (any brand, 50 calories). Top with optional low-fat or nonfat sour cream.

> **Combine unlimited mixed lettuce and other raw vegetables with 2 tablespoons of reduced-calorie salad dressing or 1 tablespoon of regular salad dressing (or 1 teaspoon olive oil and unlimited balsamic vinegar and lemon).

If you prefer to skip the Fun Food today, you can enjoy 1 ounce low-fat/nonfat cheese (or 1 level tablespoon of peanut butter) with your midday snack, and a baked apple (see recipe, Day 12) after dinner.

CHAPTER SEVEN

1,400-Calorie Plan

This plan is the most popular weight-loss formula for the majority of dieters on my 90/10 Plan. Each of the fourteen days has been carefully formulated to total 1,150 calories—leaving room for your daily Fun Food.

Each day, refer to the listings in chapter 9 to select a Fun Food of your choosing. The Fun Foods are all portion-controlled and provide no more than 250 calories, so that your daily totals will add up to 1,400 calories.

Although each meal is packed with as much calcium, fiber, vitamins, and minerals as possible, the caloric restrictions make taking a daily multivitamin/mineral supplement a good idea. Women may also consider a separate calcium supplement (see chapter 2).

Because each breakfast contains the same number of calories, if you're partial to a particular breakfast, feel free to enjoy it more than once a week. You may also substitute any of the lunches for lunches, snacks for snacks, and dinners for dinners. Be aware, however, that variety also provides your body with a variety of nutrients. And variety is the key to staying satisfied and keeping things fresh, so don't get stuck with a limited number of meals.

You can also turn to the 90/10 Recipe Appendix on page 281, where you will find ten additional delicious dinners that can be substituted for any other dinners on any night—as long as you follow the portions and accompaniments for your particular plan.

Even though you may enjoy one Fun Food every day, at whatever time you choose, you may not always be in the mood. The 90/10 Plan takes this into consideration. At the bottom of each day's menu, you'll notice a box that instructs you on healthier alternatives to add into your day if you plan to skip the Fun Food.

Remember to drink plenty of water (or non-caloric seltzer), and pay close attention to the proper servings and amounts for all your meals. If you find that you are too hungry on this plan or you are losing weight too rapidly, switch to the 1,600-calorie plan.

DAY 1
1,400 CALORIES

Enjoy one Fun Food at the time of day of your choosing.

Breakfast

1 serving oatmeal, prepared with water*
3 level tablespoons raisins, 1 banana, or 1½ cups berries or melon
Coffee or tea (skim milk optional)

> *Use 1 packet dry, instant oatmeal, any flavor that is *less* than 150 calories per serving, or you can use ½ cup dry, traditional oatmeal, with cinnamon to taste.

Lunch

Open-faced tuna melt*
1 orange
Water or seltzer

> *Spread 3 ounces water-packed tuna (mixed with 1 level tablespoon low-fat mayonnaise) over 2 slices toasted, reduced-calorie, whole-wheat bread. Top each half with sliced tomato, onion, and 1 slice low-fat cheese. Bake or toast until cheese melts.

Snack

1 apple

Dinner

Chicken stir-fry*

1/2 cup brown rice or couscous

Water or seltzer

> *Stir-fry 5 ounces boneless/skinless chicken breast (cut into strips) in 2 teaspoons vegetable oil until almost cooked. Add 1 cup mixed vegetables (snow peas, mushrooms, broccoli) and low-sodium soy sauce. Stir-fry until chicken is thoroughly cooked.

If you prefer to skip the Fun Food today, you can add an additional 1 cup of brown rice or couscous with your dinner (for a total of 1 1/2 cups).

DAY 2
1 , 4 0 0   C A L O R I E S

Enjoy one Fun Food at the time of day of your choosing.

Breakfast

2 slices toasted, reduced-calorie, whole-wheat bread,
   with 1 level tablespoon peanut butter
1/2 banana (or 1 orange or 1/2 grapefruit)
Coffee or tea (skim milk optional)

Lunch

Large tossed salad*
1/2 regular-size (or 1 small) whole-wheat pita bread
1/2 cup sliced pineapple, or 1 plum or 1 tangerine
Water or seltzer

> *Combine unlimited raw lettuce, cucumbers, mushrooms, carrots, tomatoes, onions, and peppers, topped with 4 ounces grilled chicken breast or shrimp (or 2 hard-boiled eggs), with 1 tablespoon regular or 2 tablespoons low-fat *or* nonfat dressing (or 1 teaspoon olive oil and unlimited lemon or vinegar).

Snack

Frozen fruit-pop of your choice (100 calories or less)

Dinner

3-ounce turkey burger (or frozen veggie burger)*

1 cup steamed green beans

Water or seltzer

> *Prepare burger with 1 slice low-fat or nonfat cheese melted on top, 2 tablespoons ketchup, and lettuce, tomato, and onion slices. Serve on standard-size hamburger bun or toasted English muffin (preferably whole-wheat).

If you prefer to skip the Fun Food for the day, enjoy another tablespoon of peanut butter with your breakfast, plus the other half of the pita bread with your lunch, and a piece of fruit of your choice at any point in your day.

DAY 3
1,400 CALORIES

Enjoy one Fun Food at the time of day of your choosing.

Breakfast

English muffin Hawaiian-style*

Coffee or tea with skim milk

> *Combine 1/3 cup low-fat ricotta cheese (or 1/2 cup 1% low-fat cottage cheese) with 1/4 cup crushed pineapple (packed in its own juice), drained, plus a dash of nutmeg. Spread over toasted, whole-wheat English muffin.

Lunch

Lettuce/turkey rollups*

1 frozen banana

Water or seltzer

> *Lay out a few large romaine lettuce leaves, and layer each with 3 ounces turkey breast, 1 1/2 ounces low-fat cheese (approximately 2 slices), sliced tomato, and thinly sliced cucumber. (Optional: Add 1 tablespoon salad dressing or low-fat mayonnaise.) Roll all ingredients in the outer lettuce leaves. Makes approximately 3 rolls, equivalent to 1 serving.

Snack

Low-fat hot cocoa (1 instant packet, 50 calories or less)

1/2 cup baby carrots (approximately 8 carrots)

Dinner

Steamed Chinese food*

1/2 cup plain white or brown rice

Baked apple (see recipe, Day 12)

Water or seltzer

> *Steamed chicken, beef, or seafood (4 ounces), with unlimited vegetables (try steamed string beans, eggplant, broccoli, pea pods, mushrooms, water chestnuts), drizzled with 2 tablespoons garlic sauce, plus unlimited soy sauce (preferably the low-sodium version).
>
> (When dining in a Chinese restaurant, or ordering takeout, request the garlic sauce on the side and use only 2 tablespoons.)

If you prefer to skip the Fun Food today, add another 1/2 cup white or brown rice with dinner and have an 8-ounce glass of orange juice with breakfast (preferably calcium-fortified).

DAY 4
1,400 CALORIES

Enjoy one Fun Food at the time of day of your choosing.

Breakfast
4 scrambled egg whites*
1 slice whole-wheat toast, dry (or 2 slices reduced-calorie,
    whole-wheat bread)
1/2 grapefruit
Coffee or tea (skim milk optional)

> *Scramble egg whites with 1 slice low-fat cheese and chopped
> tomatoes. (Use nonstick cooking spray.)

Lunch
Stuffed pita pocket*
Large pickle
Water or seltzer

> *Mix chopped lettuce, tomato, cucumbers, raw mushrooms,
> onion, 1/2 cup of any type of beans (or 1 1/2 ounces shred-
> ded, low-fat cheese), with 1 tablespoon of any low-fat dress-
> ing. Stuff into a whole-wheat pita bread.

Snack
Apple or pear

Dinner

4-ounce lean steak or hamburger or turkey burger*

1 cup sautéed spinach, broccoli, green beans, or cauliflower**

1/4 cantaloupe or 1 1/2 cups whole strawberries

Water or seltzer

> *Prepare preferred meat with 2 tablespoons ketchup, or barbecue or steak sauce.

> **Sauté vegetables with 2 teaspoons olive oil, and garlic.

If you prefer to skip the Fun Food today, enjoy a medium-size baked potato (about 7 ounces) with 2 level teaspoons of a reduced-calorie, soft-tub margarine or 1 level tablespoon of reduced-fat sour cream with dinner.

DAY 5
1,400 CALORIES

Enjoy one Fun Food at the time of day of your choosing.

Breakfast
1 cup dry cereal*
1 cup skim or 1% milk
1/2 banana or 2 tablespoons raisins
Coffee or tea (skim milk optional)

> *Choose a cereal variety with more than 3 grams of fiber
> and less than 120 calories per 3/4–1-cup serving, such as
> Bran Flakes®, Kashi to Good Friends®, Cheerios®, Total®,
> or All-Bran®.

Lunch
1 bowl chicken noodle, vegetable, or minestrone soup
    (approximately 2 cups)
1 small whole-wheat pita bread, 1 slice whole-wheat bread,
    or 2 slices reduced-calorie, whole-wheat bread
Water or seltzer

Snack
2 tablespoons hummus
4 saltine-type crackers, or 10 Air Crisps® crackers

Dinner

Egg-white omelet*

1/2 medium-size bagel**

1 frozen fruit-pop (any type less than 80 calories)

Water or seltzer

> *Use 5 egg whites, or 1 cup egg substitute, with spinach, mushrooms, onions, and 1 slice low-fat cheese or 1 rounded tablespoon of feta cheese. (Use nonstick cooking spray.)

> **Top bagel with 1 teaspoon margarine or butter, or 2 teaspoons of a reduced-fat spread.

If you prefer to skip the Fun Food today, enjoy the other half of the bagel with 1 teaspoon margarine or butter (or 2 teaspoons of a reduced-fat spread) with your dinner.

DAY 6
1,400 CALORIES

Enjoy one Fun Food at the time of day of your choosing.

Breakfast

1 frozen whole-grain waffle*
1/2 cup berries or sliced peaches (fresh, or canned in extra-light syrup)
Coffee or tea (skim milk optional)

> *Any waffle brand 120 calories or less (and preferably calcium-fortified), topped with 1/2 cup nonfat plain or flavored yogurt.

Lunch

1 cup 1% low-fat cottage cheese*
1/2 cantaloupe (or 1 cup of seasonal fresh fruit salad)
Water or seltzer

> *Mix cottage cheese with 2 tablespoons of wheat germ or low-fat granola (or other crunchy cereal). The fruit can also be mixed in with the cereal and cottage cheese.

Snack

1 granola bar or cereal bar (any bar 100 calories or less)

Dinner

Lettuce and tomato salad*

6 ounces grilled salmon**

1 cup steamed zucchini, broccoli, or spinach

1/2 grapefruit

Water or seltzer

> *Drizzle lettuce and tomato with 1 teaspoon olive oil and unlimited balsamic vinegar (or 2 tablespoons low-fat dressing or 1 tablespoon of any type of regular dressing).

> **Prepare salmon (or 6 ounces of any other type of fish) with 1 teaspoon olive oil and fresh lemon. Season to taste.

If you prefer to skip the Fun Food today, add to dinner a medium-size sweet potato (about 7 ounces), with 1 teaspoon margarine or butter (or 2 teaspoons of a reduced-calorie spread).

DAY 7
1,400 CALORIES

Enjoy one Fun Food at the time of day of your choosing.

Breakfast

1 cup (8-ounce container) nonfat flavored yogurt*
Coffee or tea (skim milk optional)

*Mix yogurt with 1/4 cup (or 4 tablespoons) low-fat granola cereal.

Lunch

Turkey breast or lean ham sandwich*
1 orange
Water or seltzer

*Take 2 slices reduced-calorie, whole-wheat bread and layer with 3 ounces turkey breast or lean ham, 1 slice low-fat cheese, and lettuce, tomato, and mustard. (Optional: Add 1 tablespoon low-fat mayonnaise.)

Snack

1 1/2 cups baby carrots (approximately 24 carrots)

Dinner

Tossed salad*

Spinach lasagna**

Water or seltzer

*Toss lettuce, tomato, carrots, peppers, and onions, with 1 teaspoon olive oil and unlimited lemon or vinegar (or 2 tablespoons low-fat dressing).

**This recipe yields 12 servings. The appropriate portion size is 1/12 of the entire lasagna. Cut into 12 servings and individually freeze remaining portions for future dinners.

2 10–12-ounce boxes frozen spinach (or broccoli), chopped

2 pounds low-fat ricotta cheese

1 whole egg plus 2 egg whites

3/4 teaspoon pepper

Garlic to taste

Basil to taste

1/2 tablespoon oregano

4 cups skim-milk mozzarella cheese, shredded

Nonstick cooking spray

1 32-ounce jar of tomato/marinara sauce (any brand 50 calories or less per 1/2-cup serving)

1 16-ounce package lasagna noodles, uncooked

1 cup water (for cooking only)

Cook and drain spinach well, then set aside. Mix together ricotta cheese, eggs, pepper, garlic, basil, oregano, and only half of the mozzarella cheese. Add in spinach and mix again thoroughly. Coat lasagna pan with nonstick spray and preheat oven to 350°F.

Cover bottom of pan with tomato sauce and place down a layer of the uncooked lasagna noodles. Next, spread half of the spinach/cheese mixture evenly on top, and repeat the layers (noodles and then the remaining spinach/cheese mixture). Place one more layer of noodles on top (total of 3 noodle layers) and pour on the remaining tomato sauce. Sprinkle on the other half of the mozzarella cheese. Last, pour the water around the edge of the pan (this will cook the noodles) and cover tightly with aluminum foil. Bake for 1 hour and 15 minutes, until bubbling.

Let stand to cool for 15 minutes before slicing. Remember that one serving equals 1/12 of the entire lasagna.

If you prefer to skip the Fun Food today, you can have an extra 1/2 slice of spinach lasagna with your dinner, and 1 orange or 1 peach at any point in your day.

DAY 8
1,400 CALORIES

Enjoy one Fun Food at the time of day of your choosing.

Breakfast
Chunky apple oatmeal*

Coffee or tea (skim milk optional)

> *Take 1 serving of dry oatmeal (1/2 cup) or 1 packet of instant oatmeal (regular flavor) and cook as directed. Next, peel and cut an apple into small bite-size pieces and mix throughout the cooked oatmeal. Sprinkle on 1 tablespoon brown sugar (optional: cinnamon) and microwave for approximately 1 minute.

Lunch
1 regular-size, whole-wheat pita bread

1/4 cup hummus

Large tossed or chopped salad*

Water or seltzer

> *Mix lettuce and assorted raw vegetables with 1 teaspoon olive oil and unlimited fresh lemon. Salt and pepper to taste.

Snack
1 cup nonfat pudding, any flavor (can be bought preprepared; if made from scratch, use skim or 1% milk)

Dinner

4-ounce lean flank or sirloin steak*

1/2 cup brown rice or couscous

1 cup steamed asparagus

Water or seltzer

*Marinate steak in 3 tablespoons teriyaki sauce (preferably low-sodium), then grill or broil.

If you prefer to skip your Fun Food today, you can enjoy an additional 2 ounces of steak with dinner (totaling 6 ounces) and an extra 1/4 cup of hummus with lunch (totaling 1/2 cup).

DAY 9
1,400 CALORIES

Enjoy one Fun Food at the time of day of your choosing.

Breakfast
1 medium (or 2 small) pancake(s)*
Coffee or tea (skim milk optional)

> *Top pancakes with 1/2 banana (sliced) or 1/2 cup of any other fresh fruit, and 2 tablespoons reduced-calorie light syrup (or 1 tablespoon regular syrup).

Lunch
Fresh tossed salad*
1 small whole-wheat pita bread, or 2 slices reduced-calorie, whole-wheat bread
Water or seltzer

> *Toss together unlimited raw vegetables (try lettuce, mushrooms, onions, cucumbers, tomatoes, carrots, broccoli). Add 1/2 cup cooked red kidney beans and 1/4 cup low-fat cottage cheese, with 1 tablespoon of any type salad dressing (or 2 tablespoons reduced-fat salad dressing, or 2 teaspoons olive oil and unlimited balsamic vinegar).

Snack

1½ cups fresh, whole strawberries (or ½ cup peaches canned in extra-light syrup)

2 rounded tablespoons reduced-calorie whipped cream (such as Light Cool Whip®)

Dinner

Shrimp and pasta primavera*

Water or seltzer

> *Sauté ½ cup zucchini (cut into 1-inch rounds), with ½ cup sliced mushrooms and 1 clove of fresh garlic, in 2 teaspoons olive oil. Add 5 ounces cooked shrimp (or 3 ounces salmon or 3 ounces chicken breast) and ½ cup low-sodium chicken broth to sautéed vegetables; season with basil and oregano. Pour over 1 cup cooked spaghetti or linguini (preferably whole-wheat).

If you prefer to skip the Fun Food today, you can add an 8-ounce glass of orange juice with your breakfast (preferably calcium-fortified), plus an additional ½ cup spaghetti with your dinner (totaling 1½ cups).

DAY 10
1,400 CALORIES

Enjoy one Fun Food at the time of day of your choosing.

Breakfast

Fruit smoothie*

Coffee or tea (skim milk optional)

> *Blend together 1/2–3/4 cup plain or vanilla nonfat yogurt, 1/2 cup skim milk, 1/2 cup orange juice, 1/2 banana, 1/2 cup whole strawberries (or 1/4 cup sliced), and ice as desired.

Lunch

Stuffed potato*

Water or seltzer

> *Take a medium-size baked potato (about 7 ounces) and bake or microwave until done. Top baked potato with 1/2 cup cooked, chopped broccoli and 1 1/2 ounces shredded (or 2 small slices) low-fat or nonfat cheddar cheese. Place back in oven until cheese melts.

Snack

1 ounce of pretzels

Dinner

Flake-bake chicken*

Rosemary-crusted potato**

1 cup steamed broccoli or spinach

Water or seltzer

*Preheat oven to 350°F. Take 5 ounces boneless chicken breast and dip in 1 beaten egg white that has been well seasoned with garlic, pepper, minced onion, oregano, and salt to taste. Next, dip chicken breast into 1/4–1/2 cup crushed Bran Flakes® cereal and coat on both sides. Bake for approximately 30–45 minutes (ovens may vary).

You may also choose to skip the egg white and coat chicken in either teriyaki sauce, marinara sauce, or low-fat Caesar salad dressing, before coating in Bran Flakes®.

**Cut 1 fist-sized red potato (about 3 ounces) in quarters and coat with 1 teaspoon olive oil and 1 1/2 teaspoons rosemary. Bake at 350°F until soft.

If you prefer to skip the Fun Food today, you can enjoy an extra 4–5-ounce piece of flake-bake chicken at dinner.

DAY 11
1,400 CALORIES

Enjoy one Fun Food at the time of day of your choosing.

Breakfast

Toasted whole-wheat English muffin*

Coffee or tea (skim milk optional)

> *Top English muffin with 2 teaspoons reduced-fat margarine and 2 slices melted nonfat/low-fat cheese.

Lunch

Mexican wrap*

Water or seltzer

> *Wrap 3 ounces of grilled chicken (cut into strips), 2–4 tablespoons salsa, fresh lettuce, and 1 ounce reduced-fat Monterey Jack cheese in a flour tortilla (any brand tortilla, approximately 100 calories).

Snack

Skim café latte or skim cappuccino

Dinner

Linguini with red clam sauce*

Side salad**

Water or seltzer

*Mix 1 cup cooked linguini (preferably whole-wheat) with
1/2 cup red clam sauce.

**Combine unlimited mixed green lettuce, 1/2 tomato cut
into chunks, 1/2 cup white cannelini or garbanzo beans,
and 2 tablespoons reduced-calorie salad dressing (or 1 teaspoon olive oil with unlimited lemon or vinegar).

---

*If you prefer to skip the Fun Food today, you can enjoy an
extra piece of fruit at any point in your day and an additional 3/4 cup pasta and 1/4 cup red clam sauce with your dinner (totaling 13/4 cups pasta).*

DAY 12
1,400 CALORIES

Enjoy one Fun Food at the time of day of your choosing.

Breakfast

Scrambled tofu*

Toasted whole-wheat English muffin

Coffee or tea (skim milk optional)

> *Mash 4 ounces of firm tofu. In a separate bowl, whisk together a dash of cumin, dash of garlic powder, 1 tablespoon water, 1 1/2 teaspoons mellow-barley light miso, and fresh-ground pepper to taste. Heat tofu over medium flame and immediately add in miso mixture. Stir constantly until tofu mixture is heated through. If you choose, 2 tablespoons of ketchup can also be added before serving.

Lunch

Pita pizza*

Water or seltzer

> *Split and toast a large whole-wheat pita bread in oven. Next, spread on marinara sauce and top with 1 1/2 ounces low-fat mozzarella cheese (part skim). Add thinly sliced tomatoes, onions, peppers, and mushrooms. Bake in oven until cheese melts.

Snack

Baked apple*

> *Use Rome, McIntosh, Jonagold, or Granny Smith apple. Preheat oven to 350°F. Core apple from top to ½ inch from bottom. Place in shallow baking dish and sprinkle 1 teaspoon sugar and cinnamon (or nutmeg and 1 teaspoon reduced-calorie syrup) in center hole of apple. Pour minimal amount of water to coat bottom of baking dish and cover tightly with foil. Bake for 30 minutes, then uncover and bake another 5–10 minutes (until tender, but not mushy). For microwaves, cover with microwave-safe shield and check apple after 5 minutes.

Dinner

5-ounce fish filet*
1 small, fist-sized or ½ large (about 5 ounces) sweet potato**
1 cup fresh steamed green beans

> *Broil fish with 2 tablespoons reduced-calorie margarine or 2 teaspoons olive oil, plus lemon juice, fresh basil, and seasoning to taste.

> **Top potato with 1 tablespoon reduced-calorie margarine or butter.

If you choose to skip the Fun Food today, you can enjoy a second 5-ounce fish filet with dinner, plus a ½ grapefruit or 1 orange at any point in your day.

DAY 13
1,400 CALORIES

Enjoy one Fun Food at the time of day of your choosing.

Breakfast

French raisin toast*

Coffee or tea (skim milk optional)

> *Coat skillet with nonfat cooking spray and heat. Mix 1/2 cup egg substitute (or 2 egg whites) with 1/2 teaspoon vanilla extract. Dip 2 slices raisin bread into egg mixture (coating both sides of the bread) and place in skillet. Cook until both sides are light brown. Top with 2 tablespoons reduced-calorie light syrup.

Lunch

Grilled-chicken Greek salad*

1 orange or 1/2 grapefruit (or 2 cups low-calorie, diet Jell-O®)

Water or seltzer

> *Combine unlimited spinach leaves with 2 ounces grilled chicken, raw vegetables, 1 1/2 ounces feta cheese, and toss with 1 teaspoon olive oil and unlimited plain vinegar.

Snack

1 level tablespoon peanut butter (or 2 tablespoons low-fat cream cheese) spread over 1 stalk of celery

Dinner

Vegetarian chili*

1/2 medium-size baked potato (about 31/2 ounces)

1 tablespoon reduced-fat butter or margarine (or sour cream)

Water or seltzer

> *Use any nonfat or low-fat, commercially prepared vegetarian chili, or make your own with this recipe, which yields 6 servings. The appropriate portion size is 2 cups.

1/2 cup texturized vegetable protein (TVP)

1/4 cup boiling water

1/2 tablespoon olive oil

1 large onion, diced

3 cloves garlic, minced

2 medium carrots, chopped

2 medium celery stalks, chopped

1 green bell pepper, seeded and chopped

8 ounces mushrooms, quartered

Juice of 1 lemon

11/2 teaspoons chili powder

1/2 teaspoon dried basil

1/2 teaspoon dried oregano

1/8 teaspoon red pepper flakes

11/2 teaspoons ground cumin

1 15-ounce can kidney beans

1 15-ounce can pinto beans

1 large tomato, chopped

1 28-ounce can crushed tomatoes

1/2 teaspoon Marsala wine (optional)

1 tablespoon tomato paste

2–4 tablespoons fresh chives and/or parsley (optional)

1 cup red onion, chopped

Low-fat or nonfat sour cream

Combine the TVP and boiling water in a bowl and set aside. Meanwhile, heat oil in a large stock pot, add onions, and sauté until soft (about 3 minutes). Next, add garlic, carrots, celery, bell pepper, mushrooms, lemon juice, and spices. Cook over medium heat, covered, for 5 minutes.

Stir in TVP, pinto and kidney beans, chopped tomato, and crushed tomatoes. Bring to a simmer. Cook uncovered over low heat for 15 minutes, stirring occasionally. Add Marsala wine and tomato paste, and simmer again for an additional 5 minutes. Remove pot from heat and stir in fresh herbs.

Ladle the chili into bowls and garnish each with chopped red onion and 1 heaping tablespoon low-fat or nonfat sour cream. One serving equals 2 cups.

If you prefer to skip the Fun Food today, you can enjoy 1 cup (8 ounces) of orange juice with breakfast; 1 small, whole-wheat pita bread with your lunch (or 4 Melba toast crackers); and 1 1/2 cups whole strawberries (or peach, nectarine, 1/2 grapefruit, or 1/4 cantaloupe) at any point in your day.

DAY 14
1,400 CALORIES

Enjoy one Fun Food at the time of day of your choosing.

Breakfast
Bananas and cream*

Coffee or tea (skim milk optional)

> *Mix a sliced banana together with 2 rounded tablespoons reduced-fat sour cream, 1 tablespoon slivered almonds, and 1–2 teaspoons sugar.

Lunch
Toasted cheese and tomato sandwich*

1/2 cup baby carrots (approximately 8 carrots)

Water or seltzer

> *Take 2 slices of dry, toasted, whole-wheat bread and layer with 2 ounces of any type low-fat sliced cheese and unlimited tomato slices. Place back in the oven until cheese melts.

Snack
17 reduced-fat Wheat Thins® crackers

Dinner

Chicken or steak fajitas*

Side salad**

1/2 grapefruit or 1 orange

Water or seltzer

*Sauté 4 ounces of chicken (or lean sirloin steak) strips in fajita seasonings packet and 1 teaspoon olive oil (you may also add nonstick cooking spray). Add strips of red, green, and yellow peppers, along with sliced red onion, into pan to sauté as the chicken cooks through. Wrap chicken (or steak), and the strips of vegetables, in 2 small flour tortillas (50 calories each). Top with optional low-fat or nonfat sour cream.

**Combine unlimited mixed lettuce and other raw vegetables with 2 tablespoons reduced-calorie salad dressing or 1 tablespoon regular salad dressing (or 1 teaspoon olive oil and unlimited balsamic vinegar and lemon).

If you prefer to skip the Fun Food today, you can enjoy 1 ounce of low-fat/nonfat cheese (or 1 level tablespoon of peanut butter) with your midday snack, and a baked apple (see recipe, Day 12) after dinner.

1,600-Calorie Plan

For those of you who exercise consistently, or who have a substantial amount of weight to lose, the 1,600-calorie plan could work well. Furthermore, this fourteen-day weight-loss plan is the appropriate choice for most all male dieters. Each of the fourteen days has been carefully formulated to total 1,350 calories—leaving room for your daily Fun Food.

Each day, refer to the listings in chapter 9 to select a Fun Food of your choosing. The Fun Foods are all portion-controlled and provide no more than 250 calories, so that your daily totals will add up to 1,600 calories.

Although each meal is packed with as much calcium, fiber, vitamins, and minerals as possible, the caloric restrictions make taking a daily multivitamin/mineral supplement a good idea. Women may also consider a separate calcium supplement (see chapter 2).

Like the other two plans in the book, each breakfast contains the same number of calories, so if you're partial to a particular breakfast, feel free to enjoy it more than once a week. You may also substitute any of the lunches for lunches, snacks for snacks, and dinners for dinners. Be aware, however, that variety provides your body with a variety of nutrients. Variety is also the key to staying satisfied and keeping things fresh, so don't get stuck with a limited number of meals.

You can also turn to the 90/10 Recipe Appendix on page 281, where you will find ten additional delicious dinners that can be substituted for any other dinners on any night—as long as you follow the portions and accompaniments for your particular plan.

Although you're free to enjoy one Fun Food every day, at whatever time you choose, you may not always be in the mood. The 90/10 Plan takes this into consideration. Each day you may substitute a healthier alternative for the Fun Food simply by following the instructions in the box at the end of each day's menu.

Remember to drink plenty of water (or non-caloric seltzer), and pay close attention to the portions listed. If you do not notice a difference in your size or weight after a week, switch to the 1,400-calorie plan (chapter 7).

DAY 1
1,600 CALORIES

Enjoy one Fun Food at the time of day of your choosing.

Breakfast

1 serving oatmeal, prepared with water*

3 level tablespoons raisins, 1 banana, or 1 1/2 cups berries or melon

Coffee or tea (skim milk optional)

> *Use 1 packet dry, instant oatmeal, any flavor that is *less* than
> 150 calories per serving, or you can use 1/2 cup dry, tradi-
> tional oatmeal, with cinnamon to taste.

Lunch

Open-faced tuna melt*

1 orange

Water or seltzer

> *Spread 6–7-ounce can of water-packed tuna (mixed with
> 1 level tablespoon low-fat mayonnaise) over 2 slices toasted,
> reduced-calorie, whole-wheat bread. Top each half with
> sliced tomato, onion, and 1 slice low-fat cheese. Bake or
> toast until cheese melts.

Snack

8-ounce container of nonfat flavored yogurt

Dinner

Chicken stir-fry*

1 cup brown rice or couscous

Water or seltzer

> *Stir-fry 5 ounces boneless/skinless chicken breast (cut into strips) in 2 teaspoons vegetable oil until almost cooked. Add 1 cup mixed vegetables (snow peas, mushrooms, broccoli) and low-sodium soy sauce. Stir-fry until chicken is thoroughly cooked.

If you prefer to skip the Fun Food today, you can add 3–4 tablespoons of low-fat granola cereal (or wheat germ or other crunchy cereal) with your midday yogurt snack, plus another 1/2 cup of brown rice or couscous with your dinner (for a total of 1 1/2 cups).

DAY 2
1,600 CALORIES

Enjoy one Fun Food at the time of day of your choosing.

Breakfast

2 slices toasted, reduced-calorie, whole-wheat bread,
    with 1 level tablespoon peanut butter
1/2 banana (or 1 orange or 1/2 grapefruit)
Coffee or tea (skim milk optional)

Lunch

Large tossed salad*
1/2 regular-size (or 1 small) whole-wheat pita bread
1/2 cup sliced pineapple, or 1 plum or 1 tangerine
Water or seltzer

> *Combine unlimited raw lettuce, cucumbers, mushrooms, carrots, tomatoes, onions, and peppers, topped with 4 ounces grilled chicken breast or shrimp (or 2 hard-boiled eggs), with 2 tablespoons regular dressing (any type) *or* 4 tablespoons low-fat or nonfat dressing (or 2 teaspoons olive oil and unlimited lemon or vinegar).

Snack

Small soft-serve frozen yogurt (or any frozen fruit-pop less than
    150 calories)

Dinner

5-ounce turkey burger (or 2 frozen veggie burgers, approximately
100 calories each)*

1 cup steamed green beans

Water or seltzer

*Prepare burger with 1 slice low-fat or nonfat cheese melted
on top, 2 tablespoons ketchup, and lettuce, tomato, and onion
slices. Serve on standard-size hamburger bun or toasted
English muffin (preferably whole-wheat).

*If you prefer to skip the Fun Food for the day, enjoy another
tablespoon of peanut butter with your breakfast, plus the
other half of the pita bread with your lunch, and a piece of
fruit (1/2 cup grapes, peach, apple, orange, 1/2 banana, or 1/2
mango) at any point in your day.*

DAY 3
1,600 CALORIES

Enjoy one Fun Food at the time of day of your choosing.

Breakfast
English muffin Hawaiian-style*
Coffee or tea with skim milk

> *Combine 1/3 cup low-fat ricotta cheese (or 1/2 cup 1% low-fat cottage cheese) with 1/4 cup crushed pineapple (packed in its own juice), drained, plus a dash of nutmeg. Spread over toasted, whole-wheat English muffin.

Lunch
Lettuce/turkey rollups*
5 crackers (any type)
1 frozen banana
Water or seltzer

> *Lay out a few large romaine lettuce leaves and layer each with 3 ounces turkey breast, 1 1/2 ounces low-fat cheese (approximately 2 slices), sliced tomato, and thinly sliced cucumber. (Optional: Add 1 tablespoon salad dressing or low-fat mayonnaise.) Roll all ingredients in the outer lettuce leaves. Makes approximately 3 rolls, which is equivalent to 1 serving.

Snack

Low-fat hot cocoa (1 instant packet, 50 calories or less)

1 slice whole-wheat toast (or 2 slices reduced-calorie bread
or a mini bagel) with 1 teaspoon fruit spread

Dinner

Steamed Chinese food*

3/4 cup plain white or brown rice

Baked apple (see recipe, Day 12)

Water or seltzer

*Steamed chicken, beef, or seafood (4 ounces), with unlimited vegetables (try steamed string beans, eggplant, broccoli, pea pods, mushrooms, water chestnuts), drizzled with 2 tablespoons garlic sauce, plus unlimited soy sauce (preferably the low-sodium version).

(When dining in a Chinese restaurant, or ordering takeout, request the garlic sauce on the side and use only 2 tablespoons.)

If you prefer to skip the Fun Food today, add another 1/2 cup white or brown rice with dinner and have an 8-ounce glass of orange juice with breakfast (preferably calcium-fortified).

DAY 4
1,600 CALORIES

Enjoy one Fun Food at the time of day of your choosing.

Breakfast
4 scrambled egg whites*

1 slice whole-wheat toast, dry (or 2 slices reduced-calorie, whole-wheat bread)

1/2 grapefruit

Coffee or tea (skim milk optional)

> *Scramble egg whites with 1 slice low-fat cheese and chopped tomatoes. (Use nonstick cooking spray.)

Lunch
Stuffed pita pocket*

1 cup baby carrots (approximately 16 carrots)

Large pickle

Water or seltzer

> *Mix chopped lettuce, tomato, cucumbers, raw mushrooms, onion, 1/2 cup of any type of beans (or 11/2 ounces shredded, low-fat cheese), with 1 tablespoon of any low-fat dressing. Stuff into a whole-wheat pita bread.

Snack

Apple or pear

1 slice low-fat cheese

Dinner

6-ounce lean steak, or hamburger or turkey burger*

1 cup sautéed spinach, broccoli, green beans, or cauliflower**

1/4 cantaloupe or 1 1/2 cups whole strawberries

Water or seltzer

> *Prepare preferred meat with 2 tablespoons ketchup, or barbecue or steak sauce.

> **Sauté vegetables with 2 teaspoons olive oil, and garlic.

If you prefer to skip the Fun Food today, enjoy a medium-size baked potato (about 7 ounces) with 2 level teaspoons of a reduced-calorie, soft-tub margarine or 1 level tablespoon of reduced-fat sour cream with dinner.

DAY 5
1,600 CALORIES

Enjoy one Fun Food at the time of day of your choosing.

Breakfast

1 cup dry cereal*

1 cup skim or 1% milk

1/2 banana or 2 tablespoons raisins

Coffee or tea (skim milk optional)

> *Choose a cereal variety with more than 3 grams of fiber and less than 120 calories per 3/4–1-cup serving, such as Bran Flakes®, Kashi to Good Friends®, Cheerios®, Total®, or All-Bran®.

Lunch

1 bowl chicken noodle, vegetable, or minestrone soup (approximately 2 cups)

1 regular-size, whole-wheat pita bread, or 1 serving (24) Air Crisps® crackers, or 10 saltines, or 1 serving (18) reduced-fat Wheat Thins® crackers

Water or seltzer

Snack

3 tablespoons hummus

1 small, whole-wheat pita bread

Dinner

Egg-white omelet*

1/2 medium-size bagel**

1 frozen fruit-pop (any type less than 80 calories)

Water or seltzer

*Use 5 egg whites, or 1 cup egg substitute, with spinach, mushrooms, onions, and 1 slice low-fat cheese or 1 rounded tablespoon of feta cheese. (Use nonstick cooking spray.)

**Top bagel with 1 teaspoon margarine or butter, or 2 teaspoons of a reduced-fat spread.

If you prefer to skip the Fun Food today, enjoy the other half of the bagel with 1 teaspoon butter or margarine (or 2 teaspoons reduced-fat spread) with your dinner.

DAY 6
1,600 CALORIES

Enjoy one Fun Food at the time of day of your choosing.

Breakfast

1 frozen whole-grain waffle*

1/2 cup berries or sliced peaches (fresh, or canned in extra-light syrup)

Coffee or tea (skim milk optional)

> *Any waffle brand 120 calories or less (and preferably calcium-fortified), topped with 1/2 cup nonfat plain or flavored yogurt.

Lunch

1 cup 1% low-fat cottage cheese*

1/2 cantaloupe (or 1 cup of seasonal fresh fruit salad)

Water or seltzer

> *Mix cottage cheese with 4 tablespoons of wheat germ or low-fat granola (or other crunchy cereal). The fruit can also be mixed in with the cereal and cottage cheese.

Snack

1 granola bar or cereal bar (any bar 150 calories or less)

Dinner

Lettuce and tomato salad*

8 ounces grilled salmon**

1 cup steamed zucchini, broccoli, or spinach

1/2 grapefruit

Water or seltzer

> *Drizzle lettuce and tomato with 1 teaspoon olive oil and unlimited balsamic vinegar (or 2 tablespoons low-fat dressing or 1 tablespoon of any type of regular dressing).

> **Prepare salmon (or 8 ounces of any other type of fish) with 1 teaspoon olive oil and fresh lemon. Season to taste.

If you prefer to skip the Fun Food today, have a medium-size sweet potato (about 7 ounces) with dinner, with 1 teaspoon margarine or butter (or 2 teaspoons of a reduced-calorie spread).

DAY 7
1,600 CALORIES

Enjoy one Fun Food at the time of day of your choosing.

Breakfast

1 cup (8-ounce container) nonfat flavored yogurt*
Coffee or tea (skim milk optional)

> *Mix yogurt with 1/4 cup (or 4 tablespoons) low-fat granola cereal.

Lunch

Turkey breast or lean ham sandwich*
Large pickle
1 orange
Water or seltzer

> *Take 2 slices reduced-calorie, whole-wheat bread and layer with 3 ounces turkey breast or lean ham, 2 slices low-fat cheese, and lettuce, tomato, and mustard. (Optional: Add 1 tablespoon low-fat mayonnaise.)

Snack

1/4 cantaloupe
1/2 cup low-fat cottage cheese

Dinner

Mixed salad*

Spinach lasagna**

Water or seltzer

*Mix lettuce, tomato, carrots, peppers, and onions, plus 1/2 cup of any type of beans, with 1 teaspoon olive oil and unlimited lemon or vinegar (or 2 tablespoons low-fat dressing).

**This recipe serves 12. The appropriate portion size is 1/12 of the entire lasagna. Cut into 12 servings and individually freeze remaining portions for future dinners.

2 10–12-ounce boxes frozen spinach (or broccoli), chopped

2 pounds low-fat ricotta cheese

1 whole egg plus 2 egg whites

3/4 teaspoon pepper

Garlic to taste

Basil to taste

1/2 tablespoon oregano

4 cups skim-milk mozzarella cheese, shredded

Nonstick cooking spray

1 32-ounce jar of tomato/marinara sauce (any brand 50 calories or less per 1/2-cup serving)

1 16-ounce package lasagna noodles, uncooked

1 cup water (for cooking only)

Cook and drain spinach well, then set aside. Mix together ricotta cheese, eggs, pepper, garlic, basil, oregano, and only half of the mozzarella cheese. Add in spinach and mix again thoroughly. Coat lasagna pan with nonstick spray and pre-heat oven to 350°F.

Cover bottom of pan with tomato sauce and place down a layer of the uncooked lasagna noodles. Next, spread half of the spinach/cheese mixture evenly on top, and repeat the layers (noodles and then the remaining spinach/cheese mixture). Place one more layer of noodles on top (total of 3 noodle layers) and pour on the remaining tomato sauce. Sprinkle on the other half of the mozzarella cheese. Last, pour the water around the edge of the pan (this will cook the noodles) and cover tightly with aluminum foil. Bake for 1 hour and 15 minutes, until bubbling.

Let stand to cool for 15 minutes before slicing. Remember that one serving equals 1/12 of the entire lasagna.

If you prefer to skip the Fun Food today, you can have an extra 1/2 slice of spinach lasagna with your dinner, and 1 orange or 1 peach at any point in your day.

DAY 8
1,600 CALORIES

Enjoy one Fun Food at the time of day of your choosing.

Breakfast

Chunky apple oatmeal*

Coffee or tea (skim milk optional)

> *Take 1 serving dry oatmeal (1/2 cup) or 1 packet of instant oatmeal (regular flavor) and cook as directed. Next, peel and cut up an apple into bite-size pieces and mix throughout the cooked oatmeal. Sprinkle on 1 tablespoon brown sugar (optional: cinnamon) and microwave for about 1 minute.

Lunch

1 regular-size, whole-wheat pita bread

1/4 cup hummus

Large tossed or chopped salad*

Water or seltzer

> *Mix lettuce and assorted raw vegetables with 2 teaspoons olive oil and unlimited fresh lemon. Salt and pepper to taste.

Snack

1 cup nonfat pudding, any flavor (can be bought preprepared; if made from scratch, use skim or 1% milk)

1/2 banana

Dinner

6-ounce lean flank or sirloin steak*

1/2 cup brown rice or couscous

1 cup steamed asparagus

> *Marinate steak in 3 tablespoons teriyaki sauce (preferably low-sodium), then grill or broil.

If you prefer to skip your Fun Food today, you can enjoy an additional 1/2 cup brown rice or couscous with dinner (totaling 1 cup) and an extra 1/4 cup of hummus with lunch (totaling 1/2 cup).

DAY 9
1,600 CALORIES

Enjoy one Fun Food at the time of day of your choosing.

Breakfast

1 medium (or 2 small) pancake(s)*

Coffee or tea (skim milk optional)

> *Top pancakes with 1/2 banana (sliced) or 1/2 cup of any other fresh fruit, and 2 tablespoons reduced-calorie syrup (or 1 tablespoon regular syrup).

Lunch

Fresh tossed salad*

1 small whole-wheat pita bread, or 2 slices reduced-calorie, whole-wheat bread

Water or seltzer

> *Toss together unlimited raw vegetables (try lettuce, mushrooms, onions, cucumbers, tomatoes, carrots, broccoli). Add 1/2 cup cooked red kidney beans and 1/4 cup low-fat cottage cheese, with 2 tablespoons of any type salad dressing (or 4 tablespoons reduced-fat salad dressing, or 2 teaspoons olive oil and unlimited balsamic vinegar).

Snack

1½ cups fresh, whole strawberries (or ½ cup canned peaches in extra-light syrup)

4 rounded tablespoons reduced-calorie whipped cream (such as Light Cool Whip®)

Dinner

Shrimp and pasta primavera*

Water or seltzer

*Sauté ½ cup zucchini (cut into 1-inch rounds), with ½ cup sliced mushrooms and 1 clove of fresh garlic, in 2 teaspoons olive oil. Add 5 ounces of cooked shrimp (or 3 ounces of salmon or 3 ounces chicken breast) and ½ cup low-sodium chicken broth to sautéed vegetables; season with basil and oregano. Pour over 1½ cups cooked spaghetti or linguini (preferably whole-wheat).

If you prefer to skip the Fun Food today, you can add an 8-ounce glass of orange juice with your breakfast (preferably calcium-fortified), plus an additional ½ cup spaghetti with your dinner (totaling 2 cups).

DAY 10
1,600 CALORIES

Enjoy one Fun Food at the time of day of your choosing.

Breakfast

Fruit smoothie*

Coffee or tea (skim milk optional)

> *Blend together 1/2–3/4 cup plain or vanilla nonfat yogurt, 1/2 cup skim milk, 1/2 cup orange juice, 1/2 banana, 1/2 cup whole strawberries (or 1/4 cup sliced), and ice as desired.

Lunch

Stuffed potato*

Water or seltzer

> *Take a medium-size baked potato (about 7 ounces) and bake or microwave until done. Top baked potato with 1/2 cup cooked, chopped broccoli and 2 ounces shredded (or 2 1/2 small slices) low-fat or nonfat cheddar cheese. Place back in oven until cheese melts.

Snack

1 packet instant oatmeal (any flavor, 150 calories or less) made with water, or 1 serving of plain, traditional, long-cooking oatmeal, with cinnamon)

Dinner

Flake-bake chicken*

Rosemary-crusted potatoes**

1 cup steamed broccoli or spinach

Water or seltzer

> *Preheat oven to 350°F. Take 5 ounces boneless chicken breast and dip in 1 beaten egg white that has been well seasoned with garlic, pepper, minced onion, oregano, and salt to taste. Next, dip chicken breast into 1/4–1/2 cup crushed Bran Flakes® cereal and coat on both sides. Bake for approximately 30–45 minutes (ovens may vary).
>
> You may also choose to skip the egg white and instead dip chicken into teriyaki sauce, marinara sauce, or low-fat Caesar salad dressing, before coating in Bran Flakes®.

> **Cut 2 fist-sized red potatoes (about 3 ounces each) in quarters and coat with 2 teaspoons olive oil and 2 teaspoons rosemary. Bake at 350°F until soft.

If you prefer to skip the Fun Food today, you can enjoy an extra 4–5-ounce piece of flake-bake chicken at dinner.

DAY 11
1,600 CALORIES

Enjoy one Fun Food at the time of day of your choosing.

Breakfast

Toasted whole-wheat English muffin*

Coffee or tea (skim milk optional)

*Top English muffin with 2 teaspoons reduced-fat margarine and 2 slices melted nonfat/low-fat cheese.

Lunch

Mexican wrap*

Water or seltzer

*Wrap 4 ounces of grilled chicken (cut into strips), 2–4 tablespoons salsa, fresh lettuce, and 1 ounce reduced-fat Monterey Jack cheese in a flour tortilla (any brand tortilla, approximately 100 calories).

Snack

Skim café latte or skim cappuccino

1/2 cup frozen grapes, or 1 cup pineapple, or 1 orange

Dinner

Linguini with red clam sauce*

Side salad**

Water or seltzer

*Mix 1½ cups cooked linguini (preferably whole-wheat) with ½ cup red clam sauce.

**Combine unlimited mixed green lettuce, ½ tomato cut into chunks, ½ cup white cannelini or garbanzo beans, and 2 tablespoons reduced-calorie salad dressing (or 1 teaspoon olive oil with unlimited lemon or vinegar).

If you prefer to skip the Fun Food today, you can enjoy an extra piece of fruit at any point in your day and an additional ½ cup pasta and ½ cup red clam sauce with your dinner.

DAY 12
1,600 CALORIES

Enjoy one Fun Food at the time of day of your choosing.

Breakfast

Scrambled tofu*

Toasted whole-wheat English muffin

Coffee or tea (skim milk optional)

> *Mash 4 ounces of firm tofu. In a separate bowl, whisk together a dash of cumin, dash of garlic powder, 1 tablespoon water, 1½ teaspoons mellow-barley light miso, and fresh-ground pepper to taste. Heat tofu over medium flame and immediately add in miso mixture. Stir constantly until tofu mixture is heated through. If you choose, 2 tablespoons of ketchup can also be added before serving.

Lunch

Pita pizza*

1 cup baby carrots (approximately 16 carrots)

Water or seltzer

> *Split and toast a whole-wheat pita bread in oven. Next, spread on marinara sauce and top with 1½ ounces low-fat mozzarella cheese (part skim). Add thinly sliced tomatoes, onions, peppers, and mushrooms. Bake in oven until cheese melts.

Snack
Baked apple*

*Use Rome, McIntosh, Jonagold, or Granny Smith apple. Preheat oven to 350°F. Core apple from top to ½ inch from bottom. Place in shallow baking dish and sprinkle 1 teaspoon sugar and cinnamon (or nutmeg and 1 teaspoon reduced-calorie syrup) in center hole of apple. Pour minimal amount of water to coat bottom of baking dish and cover tightly with foil. Bake for 30 minutes, then uncover and bake another 5–10 minutes (until tender, but not mushy). For microwaves, cover with microwave-safe shield and check apple after 5 minutes.

Dinner
5-ounce fish filet*
1 medium-size sweet potato (about 8 ounces)**
1 cup fresh steamed green beans

*Broil fish with 2 tablespoons reduced-calorie margarine or 2 teaspoons olive oil, plus lemon juice, fresh basil, and seasoning to taste.

**Top potato with 1 tablespoon reduced-calorie margarine or butter.

If you choose to skip the Fun Food today, you can enjoy a second 5-ounce fish filet with dinner, plus a ½ grapefruit or 1 orange at any point in your day.

DAY 13
1,600 CALORIES

Enjoy one Fun Food at the time of day of your choosing.

Breakfast

French raisin toast*

Coffee or tea (skim milk optional)

> *Coat skillet with nonfat cooking spray and heat. Mix 1/2 cup egg substitute (or 2 egg whites) with 1/2 teaspoon vanilla extract. Dip 2 slices raisin bread into egg mixture (coating both sides of the bread) and place in skillet. Cook until both sides are light brown. Top with 2 tablespoons reduced-calorie light syrup.

Lunch

Grilled-chicken Greek salad*

1 orange or 1/2 grapefruit (or 2 cups low-calorie, diet Jell-O®)

Water or seltzer

> *Combine unlimited spinach leaves with 2 ounces grilled chicken, raw vegetables, 2 ounces feta cheese, and toss with 2 teaspoons olive oil and unlimited plain vinegar.

Snack

4 level teaspoons peanut butter (or 4 level tablespoons low-fat cream cheese) spread over celery stalks

Dinner

Vegetarian chili*

1 medium-size baked potato (7 ounces)

1 tablespoon reduced-fat butter or margarine (or sour cream)

Water or seltzer

> *Use any nonfat or low-fat, commercially prepared vegetarian chili, or make your own with this recipe, which yields 6 servings. The appropriate portion size is 2 cups.

1/2 cup texturized vegetable protein (TVP)

1/4 cup boiling water

1/2 tablespoon olive oil

1 large onion, diced

3 cloves garlic, minced

2 medium carrots, chopped

2 medium celery stalks, chopped

1 green bell pepper, seeded and chopped

8 ounces mushrooms, quartered

Juice of 1 lemon

1 1/2 teaspoons chili powder

1/2 teaspoon dried basil

1/2 teaspoon dried oregano

1/8 teaspoon red pepper flakes

1 1/2 teaspoons ground cumin

1 15-ounce can kidney beans

1 15-ounce can pinto beans

1 large tomato, chopped

1 28-ounce can crushed tomatoes

1/2 teaspoon Marsala wine (optional)

1 tablespoon tomato paste

2–4 tablespoons fresh chives and/or parsley (optional)

1 cup red onion, chopped

Low-fat or nonfat sour cream

Combine the TVP and boiling water in a bowl and set aside. Meanwhile, heat oil in a large stock pot, add onions, and sauté until soft (about 3 minutes). Next, add garlic, carrots, celery, bell pepper, mushrooms, lemon juice, and spices. Cook over medium heat, covered, for 5 minutes.

Stir in TVP, pinto and kidney beans, chopped tomato, and crushed tomatoes. Bring to a simmer. Cook uncovered over low heat for 15 minutes, stirring occasionally. Add Marsala wine and tomato paste, and simmer again for an additional 5 minutes. Remove pot from heat and stir in fresh herbs.

Ladle the chili into bowls and garnish each with chopped red onion and 1 heaping tablespoon low-fat or nonfat sour cream. One serving equals 2 cups.

If you prefer to skip the Fun Food today, you can enjoy 1 cup (8 ounces) of orange juice with breakfast; 1 small, whole-wheat pita bread with your lunch (or 4 Melba toast crackers); and 1 1/2 cups whole strawberries (or peach, nectarine, 1/2 grapefruit, or 1/4 cantaloupe) at any point in your day.

DAY 14
1 , 6 0 0   C A L O R I E S

Enjoy one Fun Food at the time of day of your choosing.

Breakfast
Bananas and cream*

Coffee or tea (skim milk optional)

*Mix a sliced banana together with 2 rounded tablespoons reduced-fat sour cream, 1 tablespoon slivered almonds, and 1–2 teaspoons sugar.

Lunch
Toasted cheese and tomato sandwich*

1 cup baby carrots (approximately 16 carrots)

2 tablespoons low-fat salad dressing

Water or seltzer

*Take 2 slices of dry, toasted whole-wheat bread and layer with 2 ounces of any type of low-fat sliced cheese and unlimited tomato slices. Place back in the oven until cheese melts.

Snack
10 reduced-fat Wheat Thins®

2 tablespoons light cream cheese

Dinner

Chicken or steak fajitas*

Side salad**

1/2 grapefruit or 1 orange

Water or seltzer

> *Sauté 5 ounces of chicken (or lean sirloin steak) strips in fajita seasonings packet and 1 teaspoon vegetable oil (you may also add nonstick cooking spray, low-sodium soy sauce, or some chicken broth). Add strips of red, green, and yellow peppers, along with sliced red onion, into pan to sauté as the chicken cooks through. Wrap chicken (or steak), and the strips of vegetables, in 3 small flour tortillas (50 calories each). Top with optional low-fat or nonfat sour cream.

> **Combine unlimited mixed lettuce and other raw vegetables with 2 tablespoons of reduced-calorie salad dressing or 1 tablespoon of regular salad dressing (or 1 teaspoon olive oil and unlimited balsamic vinegar and lemon).

If you prefer to skip the Fun Food today, you can enjoy an 8-ounce glass of fruit juice or skim milk at any point during the day (or skim latte or skim cappuccino), plus a baked apple (see recipe, Day 12) after dinner.

The Fun Foods

Mmmm . . . chocolate, ice cream, potato chips, candy . . . absolutely nothing is off-limits on the 90/10 Weight-Loss Plan. You can enjoy your treat-of-choice, one Fun Food, every single day if you choose. This keeps cravings under control so you don't feel deprived.

The key is to make sure you're enjoying the right amount of your Fun Food each day. Be a stickler for portion size. Each Fun Food serving equals 250 calories or less. If you'd rather substitute a healthier food for your Fun Food one day, simply follow the instructions in the box at the end of each day's menu. But there's no reason to forgo the goodies if they bring you pleasure—remember, all of the meal plans are chock-full of nutrient-dense, high-quality food.

So enjoy your Fun Foods and savor each bite—there's no need for guilt. Just watch portion size, eat slowly, and learn to satisfy your mind while you lose weight!

CAKES, MUFFINS, AND DONUTS

Fun Food Item	Serving Size Per Day
Dolly Madison® Angel Food Bar (Mini)	1
Dolly Madison® Apple Crumb Cake	1
Dolly Madison® Buttercrumb® Cake	1
Dolly Madison® Cinnamon Sweet Roll	1
Dolly Madison® Creme Cake	2
Dolly Madison Donut Gems® (Chocolate)	3
Dolly Madison Donut Gems® (Cinnamon)	4
Dolly Madison Donut Gems® (Crunch)	3
Dolly Madison Donut Gems® (Powdered Sugar)	4
Dolly Madison® Koo Koo's®	1
Dolly Madison® Pecan Rollers	2
Dolly Madison® Snack Squares®	1
Dolly Madison® Spice Cupcake	1
Dolly Madison® Sweet Roll (Cherry or Apple)	1
Dolly Madison® Zingers® (Chocolate)	1 1/2
Drake's® Boston Creme Pie	1
Drake's® Chocolate Crumb Coffee Cakes	1 1/2
Drake's® Coffee Cakes	1 1/2
Drake's® Low Fat Coffee Cakes	2
Drake's® Devil Dogs®	1
Drake's® Devil Dogs® (Reduced Fat)	1 1/2
Drake's® Fruit Pies (Apple, Blueberry, Cherry, or Lemon)	1

Drake's® Sunny Doodles®	2
Drake's® Yankee Doodles®	2
Drake's® Yodels®	1¹/2
Dutch Hill® Donuts (Plain, Pumpkin, Sugared, or Whole Wheat)	1
Entenmann's® Donuts (Cinnamon, Plain, or Powdered)	1
Entenmann's® Light™ Blueberry Muffins (Fat Free)	2
Entenmann's® Light™ Golden Loaf Cake (Fat Free)	2 slices (1 slice = ¹/8 of cake)
Entenmann's® Light™ Marble Loaf (Fat Free)	1¹/2 slices (1 slice = ¹/8 of cake)
Freihofer's® Super Softee™ Donuts (Cinnamon, Plain, or Powdered)	1
Hostess® Chocodiles®	1
Hostess® Cinnamon Roll	1
Hostess® Cupcake (Chocolate)	1
Hostess® Donettes® (Cinnamon)	4
Hostess® Donettes® (Crumb)	4
Hostess® Donettes® (Powdered)	4
Hostess® Donuts (Cinnamon)	1¹/2
Hostess® Donuts (Mini, Chocolate)	3
Hostess® Donuts (Plain)	1¹/2
Hostess® Donuts (Powdered)	1¹/2
Hostess® Donuts (Raspberry Filled Powdered)	1

Hostess® Ho Ho's®	2
Hostess® Muffin (Mini, Banana Walnut)	4
Hostess® Muffin (Mini, Blueberry)	4
Hostess® Muffin (Oat Bran)	1
Hostess® Pecan Spinners	2
Hostess® Suzy Q's® (Chocolate or Banana)	1
Hostess® Twinkie	1 1/2
Hostess® Twinkie Light	1 1/2
Kellogg's® pop•tarts® (Frosted Brown Sugar Cinammon, Frosted Cherry, Frosted Chocolate Fudge, or Frosted Strawberry)	1
Kellogg's® pop•tarts® S'Mores	1
Kellogg's® pop•tarts® Snak-Stix™	1
Little Debbie® Brownie Lights	1
Little Debbie® Coffee Cakes	2
Little Debbie® Donut Sticks	1
Little Debbie® Fig Bars	2 1/2
Little Debbie® Honey Buns	1
Little Debbie® Marshmallow Crispy Bars	1 1/2
Little Debbie® Marshmallow Pies	1
Little Debbie® Nutty Bars	1 1/2
Little Debbie® Oatmeal Creme Pies	1
Little Debbie® Pecan Spinwheels®	2
Little Debbie® Star Crunch®	1 1/2
Little Debbie® Swiss Cake Rolls	1 1/2
Nabisco® Chips Ahoy!® Snack Bars	1
Pillsbury® Caramel Roll	1

Pillsbury® Cinnamon Roll with Icing	1
Pillsbury® Turnover (Apple or Cherry)	1
Tastykake® Cream Filled Koffee Kake	1
Tastykake® Cupcake (Chocolate)	2
Tastykake® Cupcake (Cream Filled Butter Cream Iced)	2
Tastykake® Cupcake (Cream Filled Chocolate Iced)	2
Tastykake® Glazed Mini Donuts	3
Tastykake® Jelly Krimpet Kreme Krimpies	2
Tastykake® Kreme Krimpies	2
Tastykake® Rich Frosted Mini Donuts	2
Pepperidge Farm® Cinnamon Roll	1

COOKIES

Fun Food Item	Serving Size Per Day
Archway® Apple Filled Oatmeal	2 cookies
Archway® Apple N' Raisin	2 cookies
Archway® Apricot Filled	2 cookies
Archway® Cherry Filled	2 cookies
Archway® Chocolate Chip Drop	2 cookies
Archway® Cinnamon Apple	2 cookies
Archway® Coconut Macaroon	2 cookies
Archway® Fat Free Devil's Food	4 cookies
Archway® Dutch Cocoa	2 cookies
Archway® Frosty Lemon	2 cookies
Archway® Fruit & Honey	2 cookies

Archway® Iced Molasses	2 cookies
Archway® Iced Oatmeal	2 cookies
Archway® Lemon Drop	2 cookies
Archway® Oatmeal	2 cookies
Archway® Oatmeal Raisin	2 cookies
Archway® Fat Free Oatmeal Raisin	2 cookies
Archway® Fat Free Oatmeal Raspberry	2 cookies
Archway® Old Fashioned Molasses	2 cookies
Archway® Strawberry Filled	2 cookies
Archway® Fat Free Sugar	4 cookies
Archway® Sugar Free (Chocolate Chip, Oatmeal, Peanut Butter, or Shortbread)	2 cookies
Entenmann's® Soft Baked Cookies (Chocolate Chip, Double Chocolate Chip, Milk Chocolate Chip, or White Chocolate Macadamia Nut)	2 cookies
Entenmann's® Light™ Soft Baked Cookies (Fat Free) Chocolate Brownie	6 cookies
Entenmann's® Light™ Soft Baked Cookies (Fat Free) Oatmeal Raisin	6 cookies
Entenmann's® Light™ Soft Baked Cookies (50% Less Fat) Chocolatey Chip	4 cookies
Famous Amos® (Chocolate Chip, Chocolate Chip & Pecan, or Oatmeal Raisin)	7 cookies
Keebler® Chips Coconut Deluxe® Cookies	3 cookies
Keebler® Chips Deluxe® Cookies	3 cookies
Keebler® Chips Deluxe® Cookies with Peanut Butter Cups	3 cookies

Keebler® Chips Deluxe® Reduced Fat Cookies	3 cookies
Keebler® Chocolate Chewy Chips Deluxe® Cookies	3 cookies
Keebler® E.L. Fudge® Butter Flavored Sandwich Cookies with Fudge Creme Filling	4 cookies
Keebler® Fudge Shoppe® Deluxe Grahams Cookies	5 cookies
Keebler® Fudge Shoppe® Deluxe Grahams (Reduced Fat)	6 cookies
Keebler® Fudge Shoppe® Fudge Sticks Cookies	5 cookies
Keebler® Fudge Shoppe® Fudge Stripes	4 cookies
Keebler® Fudge Shoppe® Reduced Fat Fudge Stripes	5 cookies
Keebler® Fudge Shoppe® Grasshoppers Fudge Mint Cookies	6 cookies
Keebler® Ginger Snaps	8 cookies
Keebler® Iced or Sprinkled Animal Cookies	10 cookies
Keebler® Rainbow Chips Deluxe® Cookies	3 cookies
Keebler® Sandies® (Almond Shortbread, Pecan Shortbread, Reduced Fat Pecan Shortbread, or Simply Shortbread Cookies)	3 cookies
Keebler® Soft Batch® (Chocolate Chip or Oatmeal Raisin Cookies)	3 cookies
Keebler® Soft and Chewy Chips Deluxe® Cookies	3 cookies
Nabisco® Fat Free Apple Newtons®	5 cookies
Nabisco® Barnum's® Animals Crackers	20 cookies

Nabisco® Biscos® Sugar Wafers	14 cookies
Nabisco® Biscos® Waffle Cremes	5 cookies
Nabisco® Chips Ahoy!® (Reduced Fat)	5 cookies
Nabisco® Chips Ahoy!® (Bite Size)	23 cookies
Nabisco® Chips Ahoy!® (Chewy, Real Chocolate Chip)	4 cookies
Nabisco® Chips Ahoy!® (Chunky)	3 cookies
Nabisco® Cranberry Newtons® (Fat Free)	5 cookies
Nabisco® Family Favorites™ (Oatmeal)	3 cookies
Nabisco® Family Favorites™ (Vanilla Sandwich)	4 cookies
Nabisco® Famous™ Chocolate Wafers	8 cookies
Nabisco® Fat Free Fig Newtons®	5 cookies
Nabisco® Original Fig Newtons®	4 cookies
Nabisco® Fudge Favorites (Fudge Covered Grahams)	5 cookies
Nabisco® Fudge Favorites (Fudge Striped Shortbread)	4 cookies
Nabisco® Honey Maid® Grahams (Chocolate, Cinnamon Crisps, Honey, Low Fat Cinnamon, or Low Fat Honey Oatmeal Crunch)	4 long sheets
Nabisco® Lorna Doone® Shortbread	7 cookies
Nabisco® Mallomars® Cookies	4 cookies
Nabisco® National Arrowroot® Biscuit	12 cookies
Nabisco® Newtons® (Apple Cinnamon Cobblers or Peach Apricot Cobblers)	3 cookies
Nabisco® Nilla® Wafers	12 cookies

Nabisco® Nilla® Chocolate or Vanilla Wafers (Reduced Fat)	15 cookies
Nabisco® Nutter Butter® Bites	16 cookies
Nabisco® Nutter Butter® Peanut Butter Sandwich or Chocolate Peanut Butter Sandwich	3 cookies
Nabisco® Old Fashioned Ginger Snaps	8 cookies
Nabisco® Oreo® Chocolate Sandwich Cookies	4 cookies
Nabisco® Oreo® Chocolate Sandwich Cookies (Reduced Fat)	5 cookies
Nabisco® Oreo® Chocolate Sandwich Cookies, Double Stuff®	3 cookies
Nabisco® Oreo® White Fudge Covered Chocolate Sandwich Cookies	2 cookies
Nabisco® Pecan Shortbread Cookies Pecanz™	3 cookies
Nabisco® Fat Free Raspberry Newtons®	5 cookies
Nabisco® SnackWell's® Chocolate Chip (Bite Size)	24 cookies
Nabisco®SnackWell's® Chocolate Sandwich Cookies	4 cookies
Nabisco® SnackWell's® Cinnamon Graham Snacks	45 cookies
Nabisco® SnackWell's® Coconut Creme	4 cookies
Nabisco® SnackWell's® Creme Sandwich	4 cookies
Nabisco® SnackWell's® Devil's Food Cookie Cakes	5 cookies

Nabisco® SnackWell's® Double Chocolate Chip (Bite Size)	24 cookies
Nabisco® SnackWell's® Golden Devil's Food	5 cookies
Nabisco® SnackWell's® Mint Creme	4 cookies
Nabisco® SnackWell's® Peanut Butter Chocolate Chip (Bite Size)	24 cookies
Nabisco® Social Tea® Biscuits	12 cookies
Nabisco® Fat Free Strawberry Newtons®	5 cookies
Nabisco® Teddy Grahams® (Chocolate, Chocolatey Chip, Cinnamon, or Honey)	42 cookies (3/4 cup)
Pepperidge Farm® Chocolate Chunk Classic (Chesapeake™, Montauk®, Nantucket™, Santa Fe®, or Tahoe®)	1 1/2 cookies
Pepperidge Farm® Bordeaux®	7 cookies
Pepperidge Farm® Bordeaux® (Milk Chocolate)	4 cookies
Pepperidge Farm® Brussels®	5 cookies
Pepperidge Farm® Chantilly® Raspberry	3 cookies
Pepperidge Farm® Chessmen®	6 cookies
Pepperidge Farm® Chocolate Chip Home Style	5 cookies
Pepperidge Farm® Chocolate Creme Pirouette	3 cookies
Pepperidge Farm® Geneva®	4 cookies
Pepperidge Farm® Ginger Man Home Style Cookies	7 cookies
Pepperidge Farm® Lemon Nut Home Style	4 cookies
Pepperidge Farm® Lido®	2 cookies

Pepperidge Farm® Linzer Raspberry Filled	2 cookies
Pepperidge Farm® Milano®	4 cookies
Pepperidge Farm® Milano® (Chocolate)	4 cookies
Pepperidge Farm® Milano® (Double Chocolate, Mint, or Orange)	3 cookies
Pepperidge Farm® Old Fashioned Brownie Chocolate Nut	4 cookies
Pepperidge Farm® Old Fashioned Butterscotch Oatmeal	4 cookies
Pepperidge Farm® Old Fashioned Irish Oatmeal	5 cookies
Pepperidge Farm® Old Fashioned Molasses Crisps	8 cookies
Pepperidge Farm® Old Fashioned Oatmeal Raisin	4 cookies
Pepperidge Farm® Old Fashioned Pecan Shortbread	3 cookies
Pepperidge Farm® Soft Baked Chocolate, Chocolate Chunk, Chocolate Walnut, or Milk Chocolate	1 1/2 cookies
Pepperidge Farm® Soft Baked Oatmeal Raisin	2 cookies
Pepperidge Farm® Strawberry Verona®	5 cookies
Pepperidge Farm® Sugar Home Style	5 cookies
Stella D'Oro® Angel Wings®	3 cookies
Stella D'Oro® Anisette Sponge®	5 cookies
Stella D'Oro® Anisette Toast®	6 cookies

Stella D'Oro® Biscotti (Chocolate Almond, Chocolate Chunk, or Hazelnut)	2½ cookies
Stella D'Oro® Breakfast Treats® (Chocolate or Original)	2 cookies
Stella D'Oro® Chocolate Castelets®	3 cookies
Stella D'Oro® Lady Stella®	5 cookies
Stella D'Oro® Margherite®	3 cookies
Stella D'Oro® Pfeffernusse® Spice Drops	6 cookies
Stella D'Oro® Swiss Fudge®	3 cookies

CANDY

Fun Food Item	Serving Size Per Day
After Eight® Dark Chocolate Thin Mints	7 pieces (0.3 oz each)
Altoids®	1 tin (1.76 oz)
Andes® Creme de Menthe Thins	10 pieces (0.17 oz each)
Cadbury's® Caramello®	1 bar (1.6 oz) or 6 squares
Candy Corn	¼ cup or 40 pieces
Charleston Chew® Vanilla, Chocolate, or Strawberry	1 bar (1.8 oz)
Charms® Blow Pop®	4 pops
Charms® Candy Sour Balls	12 pieces
Chocolate Chips, semi-sweet	4 Tbsp
Chuckles®	5 pieces
Chuckles® Spearmint Leaves	10 pieces

Dots®	1 box (2.25 oz), or 20 pieces
Dove® Chocolate Bar	1 bar (1.3 oz)
Dream™	2 bars (1 oz each)
Fruit by the Foot®	3 rolls
Fruit Roll•Ups®	4 rolls
Good & Fruity®	1 box (1.8 oz)
Good & Plenty®	1 box (1.8 oz)
Gummi Bears	½ cup or 35 pieces
Heath® Milk Chocolate English Toffee Bar	1 bar (1.4 oz)
Hershey®'s Cookies 'n' Creme	1 bar (1.55 oz)
Hershey®'s Hugs®	9 pieces
Hershey®'s Kisses® or Kisses® with Almonds™	9 pieces
Hershey®'s Milk Chocolate	1 bar (1.5 oz)
Hershey®'s Milk Chocolate	4 (1-inch) nuggets
Hershey®'s Milk Chocolate	2 snack-size bars (0.6 oz)
Hershey®'s Milk Chocolate with Almonds	1 bar (1.45 oz)
Hershey®'s Milk Chocolate with Almonds	4 (1-inch) nuggets
Hershey®'s Milk Chocolate with Almonds	2 snack-size bars
Hershey®'s Milk Duds®	1 box (1.85 oz)
Hershey®'s Skor®	1 bar (1.4 oz)
Hershey®'s Special Dark®	1 bar (1.45 oz)
Hershey®'s Special Dark®	6 miniatures (0.3 oz)
Hershey®'s Whatchamacallit®	1 bar (1.7 oz)
Jaw Breakers (Original)	1 box (1.75 oz)
Jelly Beans	22 pieces

Jolly Rancher® Gummies	1 bag (1.75 oz)
Jolly Rancher® (hard candies; all flavors)	10 candies
Joyva® Joys Chocolate Covered Jelle	1 bar (1.5 oz)
Jujyfruits®	1 box (2.1 oz)
Junior® Mints	1 box (1.84 oz)
Kellogg's® Rice Krispies Treats®	2 bars (0.78 oz each)
Kit Kat®	1 bar (1.5 oz)
Kudos® (m&m's® Milk Chocolate Mini's or Chocolate Chip)	2 bars
Lemonhead®	1 box (2 oz)
Lifesavers®	1¾ rolls or 24 pieces
Lifesavers® Gummi Savers®	20 pieces
m&m's® (Chocolate Candies)	1 bag (1.69 oz)
m&m's® (Crispy)	1 bag (1.5 oz)
m&m's® (Peanut)	1 bag (1.74 oz)
Mentos®	1½ rolls or 21 pieces
Mike and Ike®	1 box (2.12 oz)
Milky Way®	2 fun-size bars (0.71 oz each)
Milky Way®	6 miniature bars (0.3 oz each)
Milky Way® Bar Midnight	1 regular-size bar (1.76 oz)
Milky Way® Lite Bar	1 bar (1.57 oz)
Necco® Assorted Wafers	1 roll (2 oz)

Nestlé® Butterfinger®	2 fun-size bars (0.78 oz each)
Nestlé® Chunky®	1 bar (1.4 oz)
Nestlé® Crunch®	1 regular-size bar (1.55 oz)
Nestlé® Crunch®	5 fun-size bars
Nestlé® Goobers®	1 bag (1.38 oz) or ¼ cup
Nestlé® Oh Henry!®	1 bar (1.79 oz)
Nestlé® 100 Grand®	1 regular-size bar (1.5 oz)
Nestlé® Raisinets®	¼ cup (2 oz)
Nips® (all flavors)	8 pieces
Peter Paul® Almond Joy®	1 regular-size bar (1.76 oz)
Peter Paul® Mounds®	1 bar (1.9 oz)
Planters® Peanut Bar Original	1 bar (1.6 oz)
Reese's® Milk Chocolate Peanut Butter Cups®	1 package (1.6 oz)
Reese's® Milk Chocolate Peanut Butter Cups®	5 miniatures
Reese's® Pieces®	1 bag (1.63 oz)
Rolo®	8 pieces
Skittles® Bite Size Candies	1 bag (2.17 oz)
Snickers® Bar	2 fun-size bars (0.7 oz each)
Snickers® Miniatures	5 miniature bars
Sour Patch Kids® (assorted candy)	1 bag (2 oz)
Sour Power® Straws	1 package (1.75 oz)

Starburst® Fruit Chews	1 package (2.07 oz)
Sugar Babies®	1 bag (1.7 oz)
Swedish Fish®	1 bag (2 oz)
Sweet Tarts®	1 roll (1.8 oz)
3 Musketeers® Bar	3 fun-size bars (0.59 oz)
Tootsie Roll®	9 midgies
Tootsie Roll® Pops	4 pops
Twizzlers®	1 package (2.5 oz)
Twizzlers®	7 strips (from large bag)
Twizzlers® Nibs®	1 package (2.25 oz)
Twizzlers® Pull-n-Peel™	1 package (2.2 oz)
Werther's® Originals	1 roll (1.8 oz)
Whoppers®	1 bag (1.75 oz)
Whoppers®	25 pieces
Wonka® Nerds®	1 box (1.65 oz)
York® Peppermint Patties	4 small patties (0.5 oz each)

SPORTS BARS

Fun Food Item	Serving Size Per Day
Balance Bar™ (Almond Brownie, Almond Butter Crunch, Chocolate, Chocolate Raspberry Fudge, Honey Peanut, Mocha Chip, or Yogurt Honey Peanut)	1 bar

Clif BAR® (Apricot, Carrot Cake, Chocolate Almond Fudge, Chocolate Brownie, Chocolate Chip, Chocolate Chip Peanut Crunch, Cookies 'N Cream, Cranberry Apple Cherry, Crunchy Peanut Butter, or GingerSnap)	1 bar
PowerBar® Harvest (Apple Crisp, Blueberry, Cherry Crunch, Chocolate, Chocolate Chip, Peanut Butter, or Strawberry)	1 bar
PowerBar® Performance™ (Apple-Cinnamon, Banana, Chocolate, Chocolate Peanut Butter, Malt-Nut, Mocha, Oatmeal Raisin, Vanilla Crisp, or Wild Berry)	1 bar (2.3 oz)

FROZEN FOODS

Fun Food Item	*Serving Size Per Day*
Baskin-Robbins® Chocolate Ice Cream	3/4 cup
Baskin-Robbins® Chocolate Chip Ice Cream	3/4 cup
Baskin-Robbins® Nonfat Chocolate Vanilla Twist Ice Cream	1 1/4 cups
Baskin-Robbins® French Vanilla Ice Cream	3/4 cup
Baskin-Robbins® Vanilla Ice Cream	3/4 cup
Baskin-Robbins® Low Fat Chocolate Frozen Yogurt	1 cup
Baskin-Robbins® Nonfat Strawberry Frozen Yogurt	1 1/4 cups

Baskin-Robbins® Low Fat Vanilla Frozen Yogurt	1 cup
Baskin-Robbins® Nonfat Vanilla Frozen Yogurt	1 cup
Ben & Jerry's® Cherry Garcia® Ice Cream	1/4 cup
Ben & Jerry's® Chocolate Chip Cookie Dough Ice Cream	1/4 cup
Ben & Jerry's® Chocolate Fudge Brownie Ice Cream	1/4 cup
Ben & Jerry's® World's Best™ Vanilla Ice Cream	1/2 cup
Chipwich®	1 sandwich (3.25 oz)
Edys® Grand Light® Ice Cream (Butter Pecan, Chocolate Fudge Mousse, Chocolate Raspberry Escape™, Coffee Mousse Crunch, Cookie Dough, Cookies 'N Cream, Crazy for Caramel, Espresso Fudge Chip, French Silk®, Mint Chocolate Chips!, or Rocky Road)	1 cup
Edys® Grand Light® Ice Cream (Peanut Butter Cups! or S'Mores & More™)	3/4 cup
Edys® Grand Light® Ice Cream (Vanilla)	1 1/4 cups
Edys® Fat Free Frozen Yogurt (Black Cherry Vanilla Swirl, Caramel Praline Crunch, Chocolate Fudge, Coffee Fudge Sundae, Vanilla, or Vanilla Chocolate Swirl)	1 1/4 cups
Edys® Frozen Yogurt (Ultimate Tin Roof Sundae)	3/4 cup

Edys® Frozen Yogurt (Chocolate Decadence, Cookies 'N Cream, Heath® Toffee Crunch, or Mumbo Jumbo)	1 cup
Frosty Bites™ Ice Cream (all flavors)	1 medium-size serving (5 oz)
Frosty Bites™ Fruit Punch Water Ice	1 large serving (8 oz)
Good Humor® Ice Cream Bar (Chocolate Eclair, Cookies & Cream, Strawberry Shortcake, or Toasted Almond)	1 bar
Häagen Dazs® Sorbet Pops	2 pops
Häagen Dazs® Strawberry Ice Cream	1/2 cup
Häagen Dazs® Chocolate Frozen Yogurt	3/4 cup
Häagen Dazs® Vanilla Frozen Yogurt	3/4 cup
Healthy Choice® Low Fat Ice Cream (Butter Pecan Crunch, Cookies 'N Cream, Fudge Brownie A La Mode, or Mint Chocolate Chip)	1 cup
Healthy Choice® Ice Cream (Vanilla)	1 1/4 cups
Ice cream cone (chocolate, strawberry, vanilla): Baskin-Robbins®, Breyers®, Dreyers/Edys®, Friendly®, Healthy Choice®	1/2 cup (1 scoop) 1 cone (sugar or wafer type)
Ice cream sandwich (any brand 160 calories or less)	1 1/2 sandwiches
McDonald's® Vanilla Reduced Fat Ice Cream Cone	1
TCBY® Treats Hand Dipped Ice Cream (all flavors)	3/4 cup

TCBY® Treats Hand Dipped Nonfat Ice Cream (all flavors)	1¼ cups
TCBY® Treats Hand Dipped No Sugar Added Low-fat Ice Cream (all flavors)	1¼ cups
TCBY® Treats Soft Serve Nonfat Frozen Yogurt (all flavors)	1 medium-size serving (1 cup)
TCBY® Treats Soft Serve, No Sugar Added/ Nonfat Frozen Yogurt (all flavors)	1 large serving (1½ cups)
Tofutti® Cuties®	2 sandwiches

SALTY SNACK FOODS: CHIPS, PRETZELS, CRACKERS, POPCORN, AND NUTS

Fun Food Item	Serving Size Per Day
CHIPS	
Potato Chips (any brand)	1½ oz (1½ cups)
Potato Chips (BBQ; any brand)	1½ oz (1½ cups)
Potato Chips (sour cream & onion)	1½ oz (1½ cups)
Bagel Chips	1½ oz (10 pieces)
CHEE-TOS® Cheese Flavor Snacks	1½ oz (1 cup)
Doritos® Cooler Ranch Tortilla Chips	1½ oz (1½ cups)
Doritos® Nacho Cheesier Tortilla Chips	1½ oz (1½ cups)
Fritos® BBQ Flavored Corn Chips	1½ oz or 1¼ cups (48 chips)
Fritos® Corn Chips	1½ oz or 1¼ cups (40 chips)

Guiltless Gourmet® (Chili & Lime Tortilla Chips, Mucho Nacho Tortilla Chips, Organic Blue Corn Tortilla Chips, Picante Ranch Tortilla Chips, Sweet White Corn Tortilla Chips, or Yellow Corn Tortilla Chips)	2 oz (2³/4 cups)
Lay's® Classic Potato Chips	1¹/2 oz (1¹/2 cups)
Lay's® Deli Style Original Flavor Potato Chips	1¹/2 oz (1¹/2 cups)
Lay's® KC MASTERPIECE® Barbeque Flavor Potato Chips	1¹/2 oz (1¹/2 cups)
Lay's® Salt and Vinegar Flavored Potato Chips	1¹/2 oz (1¹/2 cups)
Lay's® Sour Cream and Onion Potato Chips	1¹/2 oz (1¹/2 cups)
Pringles® Original Potato Crisps	20 chips
Pringles® Ranch Flavor Potato Crisps	23 chips
Pringles® Ridges Mesquite BBQ Flavor Potato Crisps	20 chips
Pringles® Ridges Original Potato Crisps	20 chips
Pringles® RightCrisp® BBQ Flavor Potato Crisps	28 chips
Pringles® RightCrisp® Original Flavor Potato Crisps	28 chips
Pringles® RightCrisp® Sour Cream and Onion Crisps	28 chips
Pringles® Sour Cream 'N Onion	21 chips
Robert's American Gourmet® (Fruity Booty, Pirate's Booty, or Veggie Booty)	2 oz (¹/2 large, 4-oz bag)
Ruffles® Cheddar & Sour Cream Potato Chips	1¹/2 oz (1¹/2 cups)
Ruffles® KC MASTERPIECE® Mesquite BBQ Flavored Potato Chips	1¹/2 oz (1¹/2 cups)

Ruffles® Lipton™ French Onion Flavored Potato Chips	1½ oz (1½ cups)
Ruffles® Potato Chips	1½ oz (1½ cups)
Ruffles® Ranch Flavor Potato Chips	1½ oz (1½ cups)
Ruffles® Reduced Fat Potato Chips	1¾ oz (1¾ cups)
Sun Chips® (French Onion Flavor Multigrain Snacks, Harvest Cheddar® Flavor Multigrain Snacks, or Original Multigrain Snacks)	1½ oz (1½ cups)
Tostitos® (Baked)	2 oz (29 chips)
Tostitos® Bite Size Tortilla Rounds	1¾ oz or 2½ cups (42 chips)
Tostitos® Hint of Lime Tortilla Chips	1½ oz (10 chips)
Tostitos® Restaurant Style Tortilla Chips	1¾ oz (10 chips)
Wavy Lay's® Au Gratin Wavy Potato Chips	1½ oz (1½ cups)
Wavy Lay's® Potato Chips	1½ oz (1½ cups)
Wavy Lay's® Ranch Flavor Potato Chips	1½ oz (1½ cups)
PRETZELS	
Chocolate-Coated Pretzels	7 small or 3 medium-large
Soft Pretzel	1 medium-sized
Nabisco® Mr. Salty® Dutch Pretzels	4 pretzels
Nabisco® Mr. Salty® Fat Free Pretzel Twists	20 pretzels
Nabisco® Mr. Salty® Mini Pretzels	49 pretzels (2 cups)
Nabisco® Mr. Salty® Pretzel Chips	36 pretzels
Pepperidge Farm® Goldfish® Baked Crackers Pretzels	93 pretzels (1 cup)
Rold Gold® Crispy Thin Twist Pretzels	20 pretzels

Rold Gold® Rods Pretzels	6 pretzel rods
Rold Gold® Sticks	96 pretzels (2 oz or 1¼ cups)
Rold Gold® Fat Free Tiny Twists Pretzels	44 pretzels (2½ oz)
Snyder's® of Hanover Mini Pretzels	40 pretzels (1½ cups)
CRACKERS	
Cheddar Cheese NIPS® Baked Snack Crackers	48 crackers (1 cup)
Cheese TID-BIT® Crackers	50 crackers (¾ cup)
Handi-Snacks® Cheez 'N Crackers or Cheez 'N Pretzels	2 packages
Harvest Crisps® Five Grain Crackers	24 crackers
Keebler® Melba Toast Crackers (long)	16 crackers
Keebler® Munch'ems® Original Baked Snacks	69 crackers (1 cup)
Keebler® Original Club® Crackers	14 crackers
Keebler® Original Club® Reduced Sodium Crackers	14 crackers
Keebler® Town House® Original Crackers	14 crackers
Keebler® Town House® Reduced Sodium Crackers	15 crackers
Keebler® Wheatables® Original Wheat Crackers	20 crackers
Keebler® Wheatables® Original Wheat Reduced Fat Snack Crackers	25 crackers
Keebler® Wheatables® 30% Reduced Fat White Cheddar Crackers	51 crackers

Keebler® Whole Grain Wheat Crackers	14 crackers
Nabisco® Better Cheddars® Low Salt Snack Thins	36 crackers (3/4 cup)
Nabisco® Better Cheddars® Reduced Fat	41 crackers (3/4 cup)
Nabisco® Low Sodium Wheat Thins® Snack Crackers	28 crackers
Nabisco® Multi-Grain Wheat Thins®	32 crackers
Nabisco® Original Premium® Saltine Crackers	20 crackers
Nabisco® Sociables® Snack Crackers	21 crackers
Nabisco® Vegetable Thins® Snack Crackers	21 crackers
Nabisco® Wheat Thins®	28 crackers
Nabisco® SnackWell's® Cracked Pepper Crackers	20 crackers
Nabisco® SnackWell's® Wheat Crackers	17 crackers
Nabisco® SnackWell's® Zesty Cheese Crackers	73 crackers
Pepperidge Farm® Cheddar Cheese Goldfish® Crackers	100 crackers (1 cup)
RITZ® BITS® Sandwiches (Mini RITZ® Crackers, Cheese)	20 crackers
RITZ® BITS® Sandwiches (Mini RITZ® Crackers, Peanut Butter)	22 crackers
RITZ® Crackers	15 crackers
RITZ® Low Sodium Crackers	15 crackers
Sunshine® Cheez-It® Baked Snack Crackers	41 crackers (3/4 cup)
Sunshine® Cheez-It® Reduced Fat Baked Snack Crackers	50 crackers (1 cup)

Sunshine® Cheez-it® White Cheddar Baked Snack Crackers	43 crackers (3/4 cup)
Sunshine® Hi-Ho® Crackers	14 crackers
Sunshine® Hi-Ho® Reduced Fat Crackers	17 crackers
Sunshine® Krispy® Fat Free Saltine Crackers	25 crackers
Sunshine® Krispy® Original Saltine Crackers	20 crackers
Sunshine® Krispy Soup & Oyster Crackers	70 crackers (1 cup)
Triscuit® Garden Herb Wafers	12 wafers
Triscuit® Low Salt Wafers	12 wafers
Triscuit® Reduced Fat Wafers	14 wafers
Triscuit® Wafers	12 wafers
POPCORN	
Popcorn, popped with oil and salt	4 cups
Popcorn, buttered, popped with oil	3 cups
Caramel Popcorn	1 1/2 cups
Cheese-Flavored Popcorn	2 cups
Franklin Crunch 'N Munch® Buttery Toffee Popcorn with Peanuts (Regular and Fat Free)	1 cup (1 1/2 oz)
Franklin Crunch 'N Munch® Caramel Popcorn with Peanuts	1 cup (1 1/2 oz)
Healthy Choice® Natural Flavor Popcorn (microwave)	1 bag
POP·SECRET® Popcorn (Butter)	6 1/2 cups (1/2 bag)
POP·SECRET® Popcorn (Light Butter Flavor)	12 1/2 cups (1 bag)
SMARTFOOD® Reduced Fat Popcorn	5 cups

SMARTFOOD® White Cheddar Cheese Flavored Popcorn	2¹/2 cups
Weight Watchers® Popcorn (microwave)	2 bags
NUTS	
Almonds, dry or oil roasted	¹/4 cup (4 Tbsp)
Brazil Nuts	¹/4 cup
Cashew Nuts, dry roasted, salted	¹/4 cup (5 Tbsp)
Cashew Nuts, oil roasted, salted	¹/4 cup (5 Tbsp)
Chocolate-Covered Peanuts	¹/4 cup (4 Tbsp)
Honey Roasted Peanuts	¹/4 cup (4 Tbsp)
Mixed Nuts, low salt	¹/4 cup (4 Tbsp)
Mixed Nuts with peanuts, dry roasted	¹/4 cup (4 Tbsp)
Mixed Nuts with peanuts, oil roasted	¹/4 cup (4 Tbsp)
Mixed Nuts without peanuts, oil roasted, salted	¹/4 cup (4 Tbsp)
Peanuts, all types, dry roasted	¹/4 cup (4 Tbsp)
Peanuts, all types, oil roasted, with salt	¹/4 cup (4 Tbsp)
Pistachio Nuts, dry roasted, salted	¹/4 cup (5 Tbsp)
Sunflower Seed Kernels, salted, dry or oil roasted	¹/4 cup (4 Tbsp)
Walnuts, all types	¹/4 cup (4 Tbsp)

COMBINATION FOODS

Fun Food Item	*Serving Size Per Day*
Apple with peanut butter	1 apple; 1¹/2 level Tbsp peanut butter

Bagel with cream cheese	½ bagel; 1 level Tbsp cream cheese (or 2 Tbsp low-fat cream cheese)
Bagels (mini) with peanut butter	2 mini bagels; 1 level Tbsp peanut butter
Banana and peanut butter	1 medium banana; 1 level Tbsp peanut butter
Campbell's® Healthy Request Chicken Noodle Soup	1 can (2 cups)
Campbell's® Healthy Request Cream of Mushroom Soup	1 can (10¾ oz)
Campbell's® Healthy Request Hearty Chicken Noodle Soup	1 can (2 cups)
Celeste® Pizza for One™	½ pizza
Cereal with banana and skim milk (choose a cereal 120 calories or less per ¾-cup serving)	¾ cup cereal; 1 cup milk; ¼ banana
Cheese (all types)	2 oz
Crackers (Saltines or Wheat Thins®) with cheese	8 crackers; 1½ oz cheese
Crackers (Saltines or Wheat Thins®) with peanut butter	8 crackers; 5 level tsp peanut butter

English muffin with reduced-fat cheese	1 English muffin; 1 oz low-fat cheese
Graham crackers with low-fat milk	2 long sheets graham crackers; 1 cup low-fat or skim milk
Health Valley® Fat Free Black Bean and Vegetable Soup	2 cups
Health Valley® Fat Free 5 Bean Vegetable Soup	1¾ cups
Health Valley® Fat Free Real Italian Minestrone Soup with Saltines or Wheat Thins®	2 cups soup; 5 crackers
Hummus with pita bread	3 Tbsp hummus; 1 pita
McDonald's® Fries	1 small order
Mrs. T's® Pierogies (potato and cheddar)	4 pierogies
Polly-O® String Cheese, Low-Moisture Part-skim Mozzarella String Cheese	3 sticks
Taco Bell® Cinnamon Twists	1 order
Taco Bell® Mexican Rice	1 order
Taco Bell® Pintos 'n Cheese	1 order
Taco Bell® Taco	1 taco
Taco Bell® Taco Supreme®	1 taco
Wendy's® Chicken Nuggets, with or without Spicy Buffalo Wing Sauce	5 pieces
Wendy's® Chili (no cheese)	1 small order (8 oz)
Yogurt (nonfat, flavored) with granola	1 cup (8 oz) yogurt; 2 Tbsp granola

ALCOHOLIC BEVERAGES AND SOFT DRINKS

Fun Food Item	*Serving Size Per Day*
Beer (light)	2 bottles (12 oz each)
Beer (regular)	1½ bottles (12 oz each)
Bloody Mary	1½ glasses (8 oz each)
Cappuccino with whole milk, and sugar	1 cup; 2 sugar packets
Cosmopolitan	1 glass (4 oz)
Daiquiri, frozen	1 glass (4½ oz)
Gin and Tonic	1 glass (8 oz)
Iced Tea (Arizona™ all flavors)	15½-oz can
Iced Tea (Lipton's™ all flavors)	16-oz bottle
Iced Tea (Snapple® all flavors)	16-oz bottle
Margarita	1 glass (4½ oz)
Martini	1 glass (4 oz)
Rum and Cola	1 glass (8 oz)
Screwdriver	1 glass (8 oz)
Soda (such as Coca-Cola®, Pepsi®, Sprite®)	20-oz bottle
Starbucks® tall latte with whole milk and sugar	12-oz serving; 1 sugar packet
Tequila Sunrise	1 glass (8 oz)
Wine (white or red)	2 glasses (6 oz each)

Exercise, Logging, Losing— and Keeping It Off

Exercise:
A Key Ingredient

Countless studies have shown that people who lose weight through a combination of dieting and exercise are much more likely to maintain their weight loss than are those who only diet.

Of course, if you'd like to tackle one lifestyle change at a time, you can follow the 90/10 Weight-Loss Plan without exercise and you will still lose weight. But if you'd like to increase your chances of maintaining that new slender body, and also fight disease, improve your overall disposition, and lengthen your life, adopting the exercise habit is a very good idea.

Simple science: Exercise helps you lose weight faster because it burns calories. Remember, for any weight loss to occur, you must burn more calories than you ingest. If you increase your level of activity, while decreasing the amount of calories you ingest, you're going to lose pounds, inches, and fat. This is a simple, foolproof equation that works.

It is always a good idea to get the go-ahead from your doctor before you begin an exercise program. No matter what your condition, age, or level of ability, please remember that exercise can greatly enhance the quality of your life. If you have a special medical concern, check with a doctor or physical therapist for exercises that are suited to your condition.

MOTIVATION INSPIRATION

Not feeling motivated? Keeping in mind all the many, wonderful things that exercise will do for you is a great incentive to get moving.

Exercise Will Make You Feel Better Physically

Oftentimes you may not even realize that the backs of your legs are stiff, or your lower back feels slightly sore, or that your body feels sluggish in general. We become accustomed to living with minor (or major) discomforts, and numbed to feeling less than fabulous. Yet after regular cardiovascular, muscle-building, and stretching workouts, your body will feel less stiff, stronger, and more energized. You'll never realize how good your body can feel until you've given consistent exercise a chance!

Each exercise session will give your body an instant boost that you will feel immediately. Then, after you've made exercise a regular part of your life, your body should feel better 'round the clock. Your sleep patterns will improve, you'll get sick less often, you'll fall asleep faster, and you'll wake up feeling more vibrant. You'll walk taller, move more confidently, and feel more comfortable in your own skin. Any aches and pains you might have been living with can often be greatly reduced. Living in a well-exercised body is a joyous experience.

Exercise Will Improve Your Self-Image and Self-Esteem, and It Will Give You a Positive Mental Outlook

Regular physical activity will help your body look more toned and more youthful, and that will make you feel better about yourself. Wearing your clothes with pride, feeling that you look great, definitely produces a happy mood! Yet it is the process of becoming physically stronger and more capable that really affects your self-image. There is a profound connection between how strong you feel physically and how strong you feel mentally and emotionally. For instance, think of how you feel when you have the flu. Do you feel confident and able to tackle any obstacle? Of course not.

Feeling weak, stiff, and deconditioned is a similar sensation. Physical weakness impairs mental and emotional health. Getting in super shape, on the other hand, produces wonderful feelings of can-do optimism and self-confidence—not only because you look terrific, but also because you *feel healthy, strong, and fit.* After adopting a well-rounded exercise program, you should feel your spirits lifted even when you are simply walking down the street, feeling ready for anything.

Exercise Conditions the Heart and Improves Strength, Balance, Coordination, and Agility

You've heard the expression "use it or lose it," and this is a great motto for the human body. The body was designed for movement, challenge, and work. If you spend most of your time not moving, your body is going to respond accordingly: muscles and bones deteriorate; balance, coordination, and agility become impaired; and the heart becomes weaker. The older you are, the more your body will suffer the effects of a sedentary lifestyle.

By the same token, the earlier in life you adopt the exercise habit, the more you will cash in on your wise investment in later years. Whether or not you exercise is a personal choice. I want to encourage you, however, to become physically active and reap the numerous long-term benefits.

HOW EXERCISE HELPS YOU TO LOSE WEIGHT

- Exercise burns calories.
- Exercise protects your muscles from atrophy, so that you don't lose muscle while you lose weight.
- Exercise increases your lean body mass (muscular weight), which increases your metabolism (the rate at which your body burns calories) twenty-four hours a day.
- Exercise improves your body's shape and makes you look tight and toned.
- Exercise cuts down on your idle time, so that you're not poking around the kitchen, using food to quell your boredom.
- Exercise improves your self-esteem and gives you feelings of empowerment, so that you remain confident in your ability to stick to the 90/10 Plan, commit to your exercise program, and reach your long-term fitness goals.

KEEP THE FOLLOWING IN MIND WHILE PLANNING YOUR EXERCISE SCHEDULE

Have Realistic Expectations

Set reasonable goals for yourself and keep it fun, light, and positive. Plan reachable short-term goals each week that will not leave you feeling overwhelmed. Think of things to do that you will enjoy, and tell yourself that you're going to have a ball. Don't plan your exercise program like a dour disciplinarian. Be creative, and fit exciting, uplifting activities into your day.

Work Exercise Conveniently Into Your Day

Unless your exercise sessions are planned during realistic time slots, your workouts ain't gonna work out. Respect your obligations to work, family, and friends.

Consider your preferences. Would you rather exercise in the morning or at night? Some people are lucky enough to have leisurely lunch breaks or afternoon time slots that allow them time to walk or hit the gym in the middle of the day.

If your weekday schedule is so tight that planned exercise is out of the question, then walk home from work, take the stairs versus the elevator during the day, and definitely plan for weekend exercise sessions.

Rise and Shine

Some studies show that exercisers who work out in the morning are 50 percent more likely to stick with it. So you may want to try getting it out of the way before the day wipes you out.

Keep It Short and Sweet

Most people have hectic lifestyles and cannot afford to dedicate hours each day to the gym. Each workout should be short and efficient. The *consistency* of regular physical activity is equally as important as duration and intensity. Without any of these three elements, exercise is simply not effective. Furthermore, people who get carried away and try to do too much usually suffer injuries or exercise burnout.

Log Your Activity

Afterward, writing down what you did is a great pat on the back. Your exercise log should be a great source of pride. Whenever your motivation is lagging, you can just open your exercise log and let your past accomplishments help to encourage you.

Now that we've reviewed all the miraculous benefits of exercise, read on to learn exactly what exercise is and how much you need to be doing.

DEFINING EXERCISE

Exercise equals physical activity. It may involve hitting the Stair-Master at the gym, joining a walking club, biking with your kids, rollerblading in the park, playing a game of basketball, doing yard work, painting walls, or doing housework. As long as you're challenging your body with some degree of intensity, you're exercising.

Most physical activity works your cardiovascular system and your muscles. For example, biking conditions your heart, forcing it to pump your blood at an accelerated rate, while working your leg muscles at the same time. Shoveling snow for just thirty minutes burns about 200 calories and provides a great workout for both your heart and your upper-body muscles. It's no wonder that you are out of breath when you call out to greet your neighbor, or that your arms ache the next day.

Cardiovascular Exercise (Aerobic Exercise) Challenges Your Heart and Lungs

The term *aerobic* literally means "with air." Therefore, exercises that require your muscles to use an increased supply of air (more specifically, the *oxygen* within air) are termed *aerobic*. Aerobic activity is also known as cardiovascular activity (or cardio) because the need for increased oxygen challenges your cardiovascular system—your heart and lungs.

When you jog, the large muscles of your lower body are continuously working over an extended period of time and therefore require more than their usual supply of oxygen. Because your heart and lungs are the key players in retrieving and circulating oxygen, they go into overdrive to meet this increased demand. Therefore, in addition to working the large exterior muscles of the limbs, aerobic activity also provides a great workout for your heart and lungs.

Ideally, aerobic exercise should last for twenty to sixty minutes, depending upon how much time you have and how fit you are. People who are fit can work longer and harder than those who are not, simply because their hearts and lungs have been strengthened enough that they can handle an increased demand for oxygen over an extended period of time.

If you are a beginning exerciser, or someone who dropped out of the fitness game and is just getting started again, ten- to fifteen-minute walking workouts are great. Exercising is like anything else, the more you practice the better you get. And the more exercise you can squeeze into your day, the better. If you have time for a ten-minute walk in the morning and another ten-minute walk in the evening, then definitely work that into your schedule.

Remember that any exercise, especially if it's done consistently, will add up and positively affect your shape-up efforts. Don't let the ideal twenty- to sixty-minute aerobic workout discourage you from doing mini-workouts whenever you can.

Walking briskly, biking, jogging, stair-climbing, swimming, rowing, in-line skating, cross-country skiing, jumping rope, and aerobic dance are all examples of aerobic activity. Some of the "aerobic" classes offered at health clubs include high/low aerobics, hip-hop, African dance, kickboxing, aqua-aerobics, and indoor cycling, which usually goes by its trademarked name, Spinning. You can also get an intense cardiovascular workout from daily activities like house-cleaning, pushing a stroller, painting, raking, shoveling, and more. Generally speaking, lifting weights is *not* considered aerobic activity.

Why Aerobic Exercise Is So Important

Because aerobic activity burns calories and thus helps with weight loss and weight management, it's a great complement to the 90/10 Plan. Aerobic activity also improves the functioning of your heart and lungs. People who do aerobic activity regularly for many years are less likely to suffer from the many serious and common cardiovascular diseases. Aerobic exercise also improves your circulation, skin, energy levels, sleep patterns, and your state of mind. What's more, intense aerobic exercise releases brain chemicals called endorphins, which can leave you feeling absolutely fantastic.

Aim for the Following Aerobic Exercise Guidelines

- *How long:* twenty to sixty minutes of aerobic activity per session
- *How much:* three to five times per week is optimal
- *How hard:* low-to-moderate intensity, or 60 to 90 percent of your maximum heart rate (see section following)

Beginners, or those getting reacquainted with regular exercise, should start with a modest game plan. In fact beginners need to shoot for 40 percent of their maximum heart rate and work up from there. As you improve, you can do more activity by going longer, harder, or more frequently. Keep in mind, though, that you should increase the length, frequency, and intensity only one at a time—*not* all three at once. Doing too much at once is the perfect recipe for injuries and exercise burn-out.

Check Your Heart Rate

Your heart rate determines the intensity of your workout. You can measure your heart rate precisely by taking your pulse, or get a general idea through the "talk test."

Taking Your Pulse: To determine your "working heart rate," test your pulse when you are active or exercising. Place two fingers (your index and middle finger) on the inside of your wrist (just to the thumb side of the large cords you feel) *or* on your neck (below and off to the side of your chin). Using a watch with a second hand, count how many beats you feel in a fifteen-second span, then multiply that number by four. Make sure this number falls within your personal training range (see how to calculate below).

The following mathematical equation will calculate your training zone (also called target heart-rate zone). Generally, your training heart rate falls between 60 and 90 percent of your *maximum heart rate* (the maximum times your heart can beat in one minute). Although this formula provides only an estimate, it's a great indication of whether you are working too hard or not hard enough.

Training Heart-Rate Formula

To compute your maximum heart rate, start with 220 and deduct your age.

Then, to determine your *target* heart-rate training zone, calculate your *lower* range by multiplying your maximum heart-rate figure by .60 and calculate your *upper* range by multiplying your maximum heart-rate figure by .90.

Here, for example, is the training-zone calculation formula for a thirty-five-year-old:

Step 1. $220 - 35 = 185$
Step 2. $185 \times .60 = 111$ (this is the lower range)
Step 3. $185 \times .90 = 167$ (this is the upper range)

Therefore, this person's target zone would range between 111 and 167 beats per minute. This means that if it's lower than 111 he or she needs to work a little harder, run a little faster, or otherwise increase his or her level of exertion. And if it's more than 167 he or she needs to slow down slightly.

The Talk Test: Can you comfortably carry on a conversation while exercising? If the answer is yes, you are doing just fine. If you're panting with so much effort that you can hardly manage a weak "yes, thank you" when someone asks if you'd like a cold glass of iced lemon water, you definitely need to slow down. On the other hand, if you can belt out a Broadway show tune to the rear seats without a problem, you need to move much faster and work a lot harder.

WORKING OUT YOUR MUSCLES

Although aerobic exercise commonly utilizes your large muscle groups, doing regular weight training is a great addition to your workout program. Weight training does not produce the "bodybuilder" look. It does not result in the overly muscular look that many women fear (and most men fantasize about). Weight training improves muscle strength and muscle tone.

For men, who have naturally higher levels of testosterone, it usually does mean an increase in muscle size—*hypertrophy.* On the other hand, women, who lack muscle-building testosterone, tend to increase muscle tone without significantly increasing muscle size. Typically, muscle conditioning utilizes dumbbells and barbells (called free weights) and various types of weight machines (usually referred to by brand names such as Cybex and Nautilus).

What Can Weight Training Do for You?
- Well-conditioned muscles can improve your posture and help keep your body in balance.
- Muscles that are strong are less likely to suffer injuries.

- Weight training tones, lifts, firms, and shapes your body—beautifully!
- Stronger muscles can help make your everyday activities (lugging shopping bags, moving furniture, lifting kids and strollers) much easier.
- Strong muscles equal strong bones, which decreases your chances of developing osteoporosis.
- Weight training can help to *reshape* problem areas such as your sagging arms and your butt. Unfortunately there is no such thing as "spot reducing," which means zapping fat from specific body parts. But, by following the 90/10 Plan and participating in aerobic activity, you'll burn *total fat* from all over your body. Eventually the fat will also come off your personal problem area.

Your Weekly Weight-Training Routine

For those of you willing to add weight training to your weekly exercise regimen, keep in mind that most personal trainers recommend two to three muscle-conditioning workouts per week that work all of your major muscle groups.

A warning here is to *not* work the same muscles on consecutive days. Leaving a day of rest in between will allow your muscles to repair and rebuild themselves. In fact, when it comes to weight training, *resting is just as important as the workout itself.* For instance, if you'd like to work all of your muscle groups on the same day, an effective schedule would be Monday/Thursday/Saturday.

Another option is to do *split routines*. In this case you can lift more often simply because you split up the muscles being worked over the week. In other words, you may train your upper body one day and your lower body the next. Or, to follow the classic weight-training split routine, train your chest, biceps, and shoulders on one day, your triceps and back the next, and then your lower body on the third day. You can train your abdominals every other day, or three days a week.

Chest and triceps are involved in pushing-type activities, and your back and biceps are involved in pulling activities; therefore, they should be worked in pairs if you want to split up the upper-body workouts. One reason people prefer this type of split-routine workout is that they can devote more energy to the select muscles being worked on a particular day.

Warming Up, Cooling Down, and Stretching Out

Remember, exercise is not risk-free and can be dangerous if you're not careful. Taking the time to warm up, cool down, and stretch—before and after your workouts—will greatly reduce your chances of enduring an injury.

Warming Up: A warm-up literally *warms up* the body. By increasing your internal temperature and preparing muscles for the activity ahead, a proper warm-up can help prevent injury to muscles, joints, and connective tissue. Warm-ups can also give an instant boost to your mood—helping you go from lazy and sluggish to gung-ho and energized in ten quick minutes.

Contrary to what most people think, a warm-up does not necessarily involve stretching exercises. An effective warm-up entails a brief five to ten minutes of *light* aerobic activity (such as biking, rowing, walking, marching in place, jumping jacks, jumping rope, or some combination of these activities). You may also warm up with a lighter version of the exercise you will be engaging in. For instance, joggers can start with a five- to ten-minute brisk walk, and swimmers can warm up with a couple of easy, slow-paced laps in the pool.

Cooling Down: The goal of a cool-down is to gradually stop the activity, allowing your heart rate, blood pressure, and body temperature to slowly return to normal. Stopping intense exercise cold-turkey can stress the heart, resulting in feeling dizzy and weak. Furthermore, cooling down properly can help prevent serious health risks for older and out-of-shape exercisers. Take an extra five to ten minutes and slowly reduce the intensity of the exercise. The cool-down is similar to a repeat of your warm-up.

Stretching: Stretching maintains and increases flexibility, which greatly diminishes as you age, unless you work on it. The best time to stretch is when your body is warm, either after you have done a light aerobic warm-up or, more preferably, at the end of your workout following your cool-down. Proper stretching allows the muscles to relax and lengthen, and it can even help alleviate some built-up emotional tension. What's more, stretching may also aid in the removal of waste products, such as lactic acid, which can prevent injury and improve muscle appearance.

Some general stretching guidelines include:

- Always get your blood pumping and your body warmed up before you stretch.
- Stretch all your major muscle groups (not just the ones you think were used).
- Hold each stretch for at least fifteen seconds; never bounce. You can still feel a good stretch with slightly bent knees.
- Only stretch to the point of mild tension—not agonizing pain!
- Ask a qualified trainer to show you the correct stretching techniques; there's a lot more to it than touching your toes.

YOUR PERSONAL PLAN OF ATTACK

Now that you know how exercise can enhance your life and level of fitness, and how it will help you reach your goal-weight faster, it's time to get down to it! Before you lace up your sneakers and hit the pavement, however, take some time to figure out what would be the best plan of attack for your very individual tastes, lifestyle, and goals. Remember, when it comes to exercise, the most important element is you. So forget about what everyone else is doing—just concentrate on designing the ideal workout program for *you*.

Take a paper and pen and answer the following questions:

1. What type of activities do you enjoy doing?
2. What are your time limitations?

3. Are you a morning person or a night owl?

4. Do you like to work out alone or with people?

5. Do you prefer the indoors or outdoors?

6. What's the weather like where you live?

7. Do you want to travel to a facility, or does the privacy of your own home sound more appealing?

8. What is within your budget?

9. Do you want to involve your kids?

10. Do you have the desire or room for home exercise equipment?

The following list represents the approximate calories burned during thirty minutes of a particular activity. Notice that the more you weigh, the more you burn, simply because it takes more energy to move a heavier mass.

Calories Burned During 30 Minutes of Activity

ACTIVITY	YOUR APPROXIMATE WEIGHT (IN POUNDS)					
	110	130	150	170	190	216
aerobic dancing						
easy	144	177	201	225	252	291
intense	201	237	276	312	348	396
backpacking	195	228	264	297	333	378
(with 11-pound load)						
baseball						
fielder	90	108	123	141	156	180
pitcher	135	159	186	210	234	267

ACTIVITY	YOUR APPROXIMATE WEIGHT (IN POUNDS)					
	110	130	150	170	190	216
basketball	207	243	282	318	357	405
billiards (pool)	63	75	87	96	108	123
bowling	144	171	198	225	252	285
car washing	105	123	144	165	177	207
cooking	69	81	93	105	117	132
cycling						
leisurely; 9.4 mph	150	177	204	231	258	294
racing; fast	255	300	345	390	435	498
eating (while seated)	36	42	48	54	60	69
fencing	117	138	159	183	204	231
food shopping	93	111	126	144	159	183
football	198	234	270	306	342	387
free-weight lifting	129	150	174	198	222	252
frisbee	150	177	204	231	255	291
gardening						
digging	139	222	258	291	324	369
raking	129	150	174	195	219	249
golf	129	150	174	195	219	249
gymnastics	99	117	135	153	171	195
housework						
dusting	99	114	132	148	164	189
ironing clothes	51	57	66	75	84	96
laundry	102	117	135	156	173	192
scrubbing floors	165	192	222	252	282	321
vacuuming	132	156	180	201	225	255
washing windows	99	114	132	151	167	192

ACTIVITY	YOUR APPROXIMATE WEIGHT (IN POUNDS)					
	110	130	150	170	190	216
ice hockey	231	273	315	360	408	471
jumping rope						
70 per min	243	288	330	375	417	477
125 per min	267	312	360	408	456	519
karate	294	345	399	450	504	573
mountain climbing	237	282	324	366	411	468
racquetball	267	315	363	411	459	522
roller skating	174	207	240	270	303	342
(leisurely)						
rowing machine						
moderate	180	210	243	279	318	378
race pace	267	315	363	411	459	522
running	246	288	333	378	420	480
(cross-country)						
running (on flat surface)						
11 min, 30 sec/mile	204	240	276	315	351	399
9 min/mile	291	342	393	447	498	567
8 min/ mile	324	375	426	480	531	600
7 min/mile	366	417	468	522	573	642
6 min/mile	417	468	519	573	624	693
5 min, 30 sec/mile	435	513	591	669	747	849
sailing (leisurely)	66	78	90	102	114	129
scuba diving	336	363	390	471	444	480
skiing (hard snow)						
level; moderate speed	180	210	243	276	306	351
level; walking speed	216	252	291	330	369	420

ACTIVITY	YOUR APPROXIMATE WEIGHT (IN POUNDS)					
	110	130	150	170	190	216
uphill; fast speed	411	486	538	633	708	807
skiing	147	174	201	225	252	288
(soft snow; leisurely)						
snorkeling	138	165	189	213	240	273
snowshoeing	249	194	339	384	429	489
(soft snow)						
snowmobiling	111	132	153	174	195	219
soccer	204	245	279	318	354	402
softball	105	123	141	159	177	201
surfing	123	144	165	189	210	237
swimming						
back stroke	255	300	345	390	435	498
breast stroke	245	288	330	375	417	477
butterfly	258	303	351	396	426	504
crawl (fast)	234	276	318	360	402	459
crawl (slow)	192	339	361	297	330	375
side stroke	183	216	249	282	315	360
treading (fast)	255	300	348	393	438	501
treading (normal)	93	111	126	144	159	183
table tennis	102	120	138	156	174	201
(ping pong)						
tennis (recreational)	165	192	222	252	282	321
volleyball	75	90	102	117	129	147
(recreational)						
walking	120	141	161	186	207	234
(leisurely; outdoors)						

ACTIVITY	YOUR APPROXIMATE WEIGHT (IN POUNDS)					
	110	130	150	170	190	216
walking (treadmill level)						
2.0 mph	78	93	108	123	135	156
2.5 mph	96	114	132	147	165	189
3.0 mph	114	132	150	171	195	219
3.5 mph	129	153	183	198	222	252
4.0 mph	147	171	198	225	252	285
water polo (recreational)	222	255	291	327	363	411
water-skiing	180	213	246	282	315	360
wrestling	291	342	396	447	501	570
yoga	93	111	126	144	159	183

Logging and Losing

Y ou're ready to roll! You are about to begin your journey toward a healthier, slimmer you. The road won't always be free of obstacles, but taking minimal time to quickly jot down the meals and snacks you ate on the 90/10 Plan, and also logging your exercise, is a powerful tool to help keep you on track. It can help you in so many ways.

Most important, your food and exercise log should give you a great sense of pride and accomplishment. Weight-loss programs work only one day at a time, so take a moment each day to review your admirable commitment to the plan.

The food and exercise logs can also help you stay organized and on top of things. You may, for example, choose to plan your food for each day in the morning so that you can better consider when you might like to have your Fun Food, or whether you might prefer to go with the healthier alternatives that day and forgo the

Fun Food completely. Logging your choices can also provide you with concrete information as to any positive or negative patterns you may be repeating day after day, and it can help you in working through and correcting them.

The logs can also reflect your most difficult "food time." Is it in the evening, after dinner, or do you get an attack of the munchies late midday? Whenever it is, that is most likely your best time to plug in your Fun Food. And you'll also be able to determine the time of the day that's easiest for you to follow through with your planned exercise. Be it in the morning, the afternoon, or the evening, it's all just a matter of finding what works best for you.

Logging your progress can also help to put your slips into perspective. After an "off" day (or meal), take the time to review all the days that you diligently stuck to the plan. Do not throw away all the efforts from all those days just because of one single food slip—no more I've-blown-it mentality. The more you are able to feel proud of your accomplishments and push past your slips, the easier it will be to commit to the plan. Use your food and exercise logs to foster good, positive feelings of can-do optimism.

FOOD AND EXERCISE LOG

You'll notice that each food and exercise log provides you with the flexibility to eat your snack in the mid-morning or mid-afternoon. Most people prefer to have this snack later in the day, between lunch and dinner. However, you may occasionally choose to eat it earlier, especially on days when you expect to have a very late lunch. That is the *only* reason it's listed twice on each log page!

SAMPLE LOG

When something looks too incredibly good to pass up, think about this:
The flavor of food lasts in your mouth for only
about one minute after you've swallowed—clearly not worth all of the extra
calories that come along for the ride.

JOY BAUER

Breakfast 2 slices reduced-calorie, whole-wheat bread with
1 tablespoon peanut butter, 1 orange, 1 cup coffee
with skim milk

Snack nothing

Lunch Large salad with raw veggies, 4 oz grilled chicken
breast, and 1 tablespoon regular dressing,
1 small pita bread, ½ cup sliced pineapple, water

Snack 1 apple, 9 Hershey®'s Kisses®

Dinner Turkey burger (3 oz) with 1 slice melted low-fat cheese,
lettuce, tomato, and ketchup, on toasted whole-wheat
English muffin, 1 cup steamed green beans, water

Fun Food 9 Hershey®'s Kisses®

Exercise Fast-paced walk on treadmill for 30 minutes

DAY 1

The journey of a million miles . . . begins with a single step.

OLD CHINESE PROVERB

Breakfast _____

_____

_____

Snack _____

Lunch _____

_____

_____

Snack _____

Dinner _____

_____

_____

Fun Food _____

Exercise _____

DAY 2

Eat to live, and not live to eat.

BENJAMIN FRANKLIN
American writer, inventor,
statesman, and Founding Father

Breakfast _____
_____
_____

Snack _____

Lunch _____
_____
_____

Snack _____

Dinner _____
_____
_____

Fun Food _____

Exercise _____

DAY 3

Cauliflower is cabbage with a college education.

MARK TWAIN
American journalist, humorist,
author, and playwright

Breakfast _____
_____
_____

Snack _____

Lunch _____
_____
_____

Snack _____

Dinner _____
_____
_____

Fun Food _____

Exercise _____

DAY 4

The first wealth is health.

RALPH WALDO EMERSON
American author, poet,
and philosopher

Breakfast _____
_____
_____

Snack _____

Lunch _____
_____
_____

Snack _____

Dinner _____
_____
_____

Fun Food _____

Exercise _____

DAY 5

Life isn't about finding yourself. Life is about creating yourself.

GEORGE BERNARD SHAW
Irish satirist, critic, wit, and dramatist

Breakfast _____

_____

_____

Snack _____

Lunch _____

_____

_____

Snack _____

Dinner _____

_____

_____

Fun Food _____

Exercise _____

DAY 6

Stand up to your obstacles and do something about them.
You will find that they haven't half the strength you think they have.

NORMAN VINCENT PEALE
American cleric and author

Breakfast _____

_____

_____

Snack _____

Lunch _____

_____

_____

Snack _____

Dinner _____

_____

_____

Fun Food _____

Exercise _____

DAY 7

I've been on a constant diet for the last two decades. I've lost a total of 789 pounds. By all accounts, I should be hanging from a charm bracelet.

ERMA BOMBECK
American author, humorist,
speaker, and syndicated columnist

Breakfast _____

_____

_____

Snack _____

Lunch _____

_____

_____

Snack _____

Dinner _____

_____

_____

Fun Food _____

Exercise _____

DAY 8

Keep away from people who try to belittle your ambitions. Small people always do that, but the really great make you feel that you, too, can become great.

MARK TWAIN
American journalist, humorist,
author, and playwright

Breakfast _____

_____

_____

Snack _____

Lunch _____

_____

_____

Snack _____

Dinner _____

_____

_____

Fun Food _____

Exercise _____

DAY 9

Never let the fear of striking out get in your way.

GEORGE HERMAN "BABE" RUTH
American professional baseball player

Breakfast _____
_____
_____

Snack _____

Lunch _____
_____
_____

Snack _____

Dinner _____
_____
_____

Fun Food _____

Exercise _____

DAY 10

An active mind cannot exist in an inactive body.

GENERAL GEORGE PATTON
American military strategist and WWII hero

Breakfast _____
_____
_____

Snack _____

Lunch _____
_____
_____

Snack _____

Dinner _____
_____
_____

Fun Food _____

Exercise _____

DAY 11

To lengthen thy life, lessen thy meals.

BENJAMIN FRANKLIN
American writer, inventor,
statesman, and Founding Father

Breakfast _____
_____
_____

Snack _____

Lunch _____
_____
_____

Snack _____

Dinner _____
_____
_____

Fun Food _____

Exercise _____

DAY 12

My doctor told me to stop having intimate dinners for four.
Unless there are three other people.

ORSON WELLES
writer, director, actor,
magician, and raconteur

Breakfast _____

_____

_____

Snack _____

Lunch _____

_____

_____

Snack _____

Dinner _____

_____

_____

Fun Food _____

Exercise _____

DAY 13

It is health that is real wealth and not pieces of gold and silver.

MOHANDAS K. GANDHI
leader of the Indian National Congress
and champion of nonviolence

Breakfast _____

_____

_____

Snack _____

Lunch _____

_____

_____

Snack _____

Dinner _____

_____

_____

Fun Food _____

Exercise _____

DAY 14

Never talk defeat. Use words like hope, belief, faith, victory.

NORMAN VINCENT PEALE
American cleric and author

Breakfast _____
_____
_____

Snack _____

Lunch _____
_____
_____

Snack _____

Dinner _____
_____
_____

Fun Food _____

Exercise _____

CHAPTER TWELVE

Maintenance: Continued Effort, Continued Success

Reaching your weight-loss goals will boost your confidence and raise your spirits. All this good cheer, however, doesn't mean you should relax and return to the way you ate before the 90/10 Plan. This plan teaches you that all foods can fit into a healthy lifestyle, and that weight management is not about deprivation. In order to maintain your new body, you'll need to steer clear of old food habits and continue to practice self-discipline and food awareness.

THE IMPORTANCE OF MAINTENANCE

Some people find that maintaining their new weight requires almost more effort than getting there. Think about it. On the way down toward your goal, your hard work is rewarded by decreasing scale numbers and smaller clothing sizes. Euphoria! While you are losing, you're striving to reach a tangible goal—a goal that helps to keep you motivated and in control.

Maintaining is quite another story. Without the emotional high that comes with the dropping digits and baggier jeans, some people find it hard to sustain their motivation. And even if you find that staying at your goal look and feel is relatively easy, one thing is for certain: it is never completely effortless. If you are going to be successful at the maintenance game, you still must watch your portions, continue to exercise, and keep an eye on the way your clothes fit. The effort to maintain your weight is well worth it, however, because gaining back the weight you lost can do significant damage to your physical and emotional wellness.

Here are some reasons to maintain your weight loss:

Metabolism

Gaining and losing weight plays havoc with your metabolism—the rate at which your body burns calories. The more you lose and then gain back, the harder it will be to lose weight permanently. If you have been a frequent rebounder, this doesn't mean that it's impossible to reach and maintain your goal weight; it just means that it will require a little more effort.

Health

For the sake of maximum health, set your goal for a weight that is appropriate for your height, age, and genetic body type. And if you are having a very difficult time maintaining your weight, you probably need to reconsider that goal weight. Many people find that their healthiest, most attractive weight is actually a good five pounds over what they believed was their ideal.

Trying to maintain a weight that is too low can lead to overeating and gaining the weight back, which is known as yo-yo dieting. Weight fluctuation stresses many organs, including the digestive system, the heart, and the liver. For optimal health, lose weight slowly and then maintain your weight loss through continued calorie control and exercise.

Confidence

Losing weight and getting in shape will increase your confidence. You might feel less shy, more sure of yourself, emotionally stronger, and perhaps more outgoing. Tasks or challenges you might never have considered in the past may now seem reasonable or even exciting.

Gaining the weight back, however, usually results in a big dip in self-image and mood. These negative feelings will not only throw a dark cloud over your days, but will also challenge your ability to "do it again." You might question the possibility of ever reaching your goal weight and maintaining it.

Having confidence in your ability to be successful at fitness significantly affects self-discipline and willpower. Don't compromise your faith in yourself by eating too much or giving up the exercise. Continued effort will bring you continued success and invaluable confidence that will improve all aspects of your life.

THE 90/10 MAINTENANCE PLAN

There are several lifestyle habits that you'll need to acquire if you are going to be successful at the maintenance game.

Portion Control

It's the number-one factor determining your weight: How much food are you eating? How big are your meals? It's very easy to slip back into the habit of eating more food at each meal. If you don't consistently watch the size of your meals and snacks, you might eat a little more, and then a bit more than that, and before you know it you've packed on some of the weight you had lost.

Be extra careful when eating out in restaurants or getting to-go food from the deli. Most restaurant meals are double the size of a healthy, weight-friendly portion. So make it a point to only eat half of your meal if it's an oversized portion. Save the other half for later, share it with a friend, give it to your dog, throw it away— whatever you do, don't eat the whole, supersized serving! If you can, order one or two appetizers as a main course, or order a half-portion or a child's meal.

Try to rid yourself of that all-you-can-eat mentality, and forget the idea that cleaning your plate equals getting your money's worth. Think of all the money people spend on diets and weight loss—it's obviously worth more to just eat half your entrée and stay slim.

And be aware that alcohol lowers your inhibitions and can cause bad food choices. So be mindful of how alcohol affects your meals. If you notice that you tend to eat more or choose unwisely after drinking, then have a glass of wine *after* they've cleared away your meal. Although alcohol is calorie-dense and virtually nutrient-free, in careful moderation it can be worked into any weight-management plan.

Remember, you don't want to stay slim by denying yourself your favorite foods, and you don't want to go for long periods of time without eating. Having small, portion-controlled meals and snacks at the appropriate times are your best way to maintain the weight loss you achieve. If you feel slightly deprived after eating a meal, tell yourself that if you are hungry in an hour, you can definitely enjoy another small snack. Oftentimes, however, you're not going to feel hungry by the time that hour has passed, and the deprivation you felt was due to emotional hunger (or boredom or habit), not physical hunger.

What your body requires and what your mind craves are often two very different things. Concentrate on how great it feels to be slim and healthy. Maintaining your goal look is definitely worth giving up the habit of noshing huge amounts of food.

Satisfaction Guaranteed

Because our fat-phobic, diet-obsessed society constantly bombards us with fat-is-evil/sugar-is-evil messages, it's easy to feel guilty for indulging in your favorite sugary, salty, fatty treats. The 90/10 Weight-Loss Plan, however, teaches that there is no reason for this useless guilt. You can eat whatever you want! Don't deny yourself! Treat your taste buds to your favorite creamy, sweet desserts!

The key to eating these rich temptations while staying slim is, again, portion control. You may choose to continue to eat your Fun Foods allowance once every day while maintaining your weight loss and satisfying your sweet tooth, or you might become comfortable with just eating smaller amounts of these foods whenever you feel like it—within reason, of course. But stay aware of how much dessert (or other fun munchies) you're eating each day and try not to exceed 250 calories—while always watching your other portions too.

Eat every treat extra slowly and savor each bite. Feeling guilty for indulging in a sweet treat often causes us to eat faster, which in turn causes us to eat even more, and then feel even more guilty when we're done. So steer clear of guilt and move in the direction of pride and self-control. Don't deny yourself, but don't let yourself eat too much either!

Consistent Exercise

Countless research studies have shown that people who exercise are more successful at maintaining weight loss than those who try to stay slim with calorie-control alone. And increasing your lean body mass (muscle mass) through exercise will help you to maintain your weight loss, because muscle burns significant calories around the clock.

The more muscle on your body, the higher your metabolism and the more you'll be able to eat and still stay at your ideal size. Exercise also lifts the mood and will give you confidence in your ability to maintain discipline at the dinner table.

Body Awareness

Being aware of how your body looks and feels is the most important aspect of the maintenance plan. Whether you weigh yourself once a week, or use a tape measure to keep track of your measurements, or just pay extra-close attention to how snugly your smallest jeans fit, keeping aware of your body is crucial.

So weigh or measure yourself regularly, and make it a rule that when the scale goes up five pounds, or you feel your clothes getting snug—you'll take action!

GETTING BACK ON TRACK
AFTER A SMALL SETBACK

Face it: you're human. You may not be able to maintain your weight loss perfectly. Statistics show that most people who lose weight gain some of it back, while others gain back all their pounds, and still others gain so much that they end up heavier than when they started.

Many people also gain back a little bit at different times, such as after the holiday season or during a vacation. This is normal and expected. A small weight gain is nothing to get down in the dumps about—you can't expect to stay perfectly at your goal weight without any fluctuation whatsoever. So allow yourself to gain two or three pounds without worrying. But, as I said, after your weight has crept up five pounds it's time to do something about it. And the key to dealing with the gain-back phenomenon is to catch it early—before the minor setback has turned into a weight gain that will affect your confidence and will take significant time and effort to rectify.

If you've not already made the 90/10 Weight-Loss Plan a part of your everyday lifestyle, and you find that you need the structure again, return to the plan for two weeks and also try to increase exercise. Experiment with making your portions smaller, and start logging your food and exercise again for extra motivation. I have provided fourteen days' worth of food logs—enough to make followers pay attention to planning and to become aware of their good and bad habits. Some people may prefer to log their food and exercise indefinitely (and they will look forward to a future 90/10 Workbook).

Try to learn something from the experience. Maybe you need to eat out in restaurants less often, or plan your exercise workouts in the morning when they are more likely to happen. Just keep at it and the weight will soon fall off again.

Whatever you do, stay aware of your body, and don't let a five-pound weight gain turn into twenty. You've worked too hard to slip back now!

Additional 90/10 Recipes

All of the following dinner recipes were created to provide you with options and greater variety on your 90/10 Weight-Loss Plan. Enjoy cooking any of the delicious dinners listed in this section, on any night you choose. Just be sure to follow the directions at the end of each recipe for your specific plan—portion size and accompaniments will vary.

SPAGHETTI AND TURKEY MEATBALLS

Yields approximately 21 turkey meatballs.

1/2 box spaghetti

1 pound lean ground turkey breast (all ground white meat)

Black pepper to taste

Garlic powder to taste

Parsley to taste

Paprika to taste

Chopped, dehydrated onion flakes to taste

1 1/2 jars marinara sauce (26 ounces each jar; choose any brand 50
   calories or less per serving, such as Healthy Choice®, Ragu®
   Light, or Classico® Tomato and Garlic)

Cook spaghetti as directed on box. Drain and set aside.

Season ground turkey breast with black pepper, garlic powder,
parsley, paprika, and chopped, dehydrated onion flakes. Shape meat
into 1-inch balls and throw into large pot with marinara sauce.
Cook on low flame for approximately 50–60 minutes.

1,200-Calorie Plan

3 turkey meatballs

1 cup cooked pasta

1,400-Calorie Plan

Salad (lettuce, cucumbers, carrots, onions, peppers, mushrooms,
   and tomatoes)

2 tablespoons low-fat or nonfat Italian dressing

3 turkey meatballs

1 cup cooked pasta

1,600-Calorie Plan

Salad (lettuce, cucumbers, carrots, onions, peppers, mushrooms, and tomatoes)

2 tablespoons low-fat or nonfat Italian dressing

5 turkey meatballs

1 cup cooked pasta

1 tablespoon Parmesan cheese

ITALIAN CASSEROLE

Yields 8 2-cup servings.

1¼ pounds extra lean chopped turkey meat

Garlic to taste

Pepper to taste

2 cans Campbell's Condensed Tomato Soup

⅓ cup water

⅓ 26-ounce jar marinara sauce (any brand 50 calories or less per serving, such as Healthy Choice®, Ragu® Light, or Classico® Tomato and Basil)

1 pound medium-wide noodles

1 cup low-fat shredded cheddar cheese

Liberally season chopped turkey meat with garlic and pepper. Brown in large frying pan over medium flame. Drain off all fat and liquid. To the meat add tomato soup, water, and marinara sauce. Mix thoroughly and simmer for 10 minutes over low flame. Separately, cook and drain noodles. Add meat sauce to noodles and stir evenly while sprinkling on grated cheese.

1,200-Calorie Plan

1 1/2 cups Italian casserole

1,400-Calorie Plan

2 cups Italian casserole

1,600-Calorie Plan

2 cups Italian casserole
Baked apple (or another fruit of choice)

SOUR CREAM CHICKEN

Yields 4 servings.

4 skinless/boneless chicken breasts (1 1/4 pounds total; approximately 5 ounces each breast)
8-ounce container reduced-fat sour cream
1/4 cup seasoned bread crumbs
Nonstick cooking spray
2 tablespoons Parmesan cheese
1 teaspoon oregano

Preheat oven to 375°F. Thoroughly clean all chicken pieces. Coat each breast in reduced-fat sour cream and then cover all sides in bread crumbs. Coat a baking pan with nonstick cooking spray and place chicken in pan. Sprinkle on Parmesan and oregano, and bake at 375°F for 20–30 minutes or until chicken is no longer pink.

1,200-Calorie Plan

1 chicken breast (approximately 5 ounces)

1 cup steamed spinach or broccoli or peapods, with lemon pepper seasoning

1,400-Calorie Plan

1 chicken breast (approximately 5 ounces)

1 cup steamed spinach or broccoli or peapods, with lemon pepper seasoning

1 apple or 1 orange or 1/2 grapefruit

1,600-Calorie Plan

1 chicken breast (approximately 5 ounces)

1 cup steamed spinach or broccoli or peapods, with lemon pepper seasoning

1/2 cup brown rice

1 apple or 1 orange or 1/2 grapefruit

CHICKEN CACCIATORE

Yields 6 servings.

2 26-ounce jars marinara sauce (any brand 50 calories or less per serving, such as Healthy Choice®, Ragu® Light, Classico® Tomato and Basil)

½ large green pepper

½ large red pepper

½ large yellow pepper

2 cups sliced mushrooms

6 large, skinless/boneless chicken cutlets (2 pounds; approximately 5 ounces each breast), cut into thirds

Heat marinara sauce in large pot until boiling. Throw in peppers and mushrooms and simmer 5 minutes. Add all chicken pieces and mix thoroughly. Cover pot and cook on low for 45 minutes.

1,200-Calorie Plan

3 pieces of chicken breast, cut up and mixed with vegetables and sauce

1,400-Calorie Plan

3 pieces of chicken breast, cut up and mixed with vegetables and sauce

Salad with lettuce, tomatoes, carrots, onions, and peppers

2 tablespoons low-fat or nonfat dressing

1,600-Calorie Plan

4 pieces of chicken breast, cut up

Salad with lettuce, tomatoes, carrots, onions, and peppers

2 tablespoons low-fat or nonfat dressing

SOLE FLORENTINE

Yields 4 servings.

1 onion, sliced

3 teaspoons olive oil

4 cups spinach leaves

2 tablespoons orange juice

1 tablespoon reduced-sodium soy sauce

1 pound sole filets

Black pepper to taste

Garlic powder to taste

Paprika

1 lemon, thinly sliced

Place sliced onion on bottom of microwave-safe platter. Drizzle 2 teaspoons olive oil on top. Cover with plastic wrap and microwave on high for approximately 3 minutes (or until onions are tender). Layer spinach leaves on top of cooked onion, cover, and microwave again for another 2–3 minutes. Set aside.

In a separate bowl, mix together orange juice, soy sauce, and remaining olive oil. Drizzle over spinach/onion mixture and set aside.

Preheat oven to 375°F. Rinse fish and place on top of the spinach/onion mixture. Liberally season with fresh-ground pepper, garlic powder, and paprika, and top each filet with a lemon slice. Bake uncovered in oven for 15–20 minutes (or until sole is flaky).

1,200-Calorie Plan

1 serving sole Florentine (¼ of dish)
1 fist-sized baked potato, plain

1,400-Calorie Plan

1 serving sole Florentine (¼ of dish)
1 fist-sized baked potato with 1 tablespoon reduced-fat spread
½ grapefruit or 1 orange or 1 cup sliced pineapple or ¼ cantaloupe

1,600-Calorie Plan

2 servings sole Florentine (½ of dish)
1 fist-sized baked potato, plain

BOUILLABAISSE

Yields approximately 6 2-cup servings.

1 cup chopped white onion
2 tablespoons chopped garlic
2 celery stalks, chopped
¼ cup olive oil
2 cups water
2 14½-ounce cans of whole tomatoes, chopped with liquid

2 cups sliced mushrooms

1 teaspoon dried thyme

1 teaspoon bay leaves

2 pounds crab (fresh crab or seafood salad meat)

1/2 pound bay scallops

1/2 pound of shrimp

1/4 cup chopped parsley

In a large frying pan, over medium-high flame, sauté onion, garlic, celery, and olive oil until tender (approximately 10 minutes). In a separate large pot, pour in water, chopped tomatoes with liquid, mushrooms, thyme, bay leaves, and the onion/celery/garlic mixture. Bring to a boil. Stir in crab, scallops, and peeled shrimp. Bring to a boil again, reduce heat, and simmer for 10–15 minutes. Stir in chopped parsley.

1,200-Calorie Plan
1 serving bouillabaisse (2 cups)

1,400-Calorie Plan
1 serving bouillabaisse (2 cups)
Salad with lettuce, tomatoes, carrots, onion, peppers, and mushrooms
2 tablespoons low-fat or nonfat Italian dressing

1,600-Calorie Plan
1 serving bouillabaisse (2 cups)
Salad with lettuce, tomatoes, carrots, onion, peppers, and mushrooms
2 tablespoons low-fat or nonfat Italian dressing
1 slice of Italian bread

VEAL PICCATA

Yields 4 servings.

1 1/4 pounds veal, thinly sliced

1/2 cup flour

Nonstick cooking spray

2 teaspoons olive oil

1/2 cup fat-free chicken broth

1 1/2 cups sliced mushrooms

1 lemon

Garlic powder to taste

3 tablespoons parsley, chopped

Paprika

Cut veal slices into 4 serving pieces and pound lightly. Coat each piece with flour. Coat skillet with nonstick cooking spray and olive oil.

Cook veal over medium heat until lightly browned on both sides. Add chicken broth and sliced mushrooms and sauté until lightly browned. Squeeze lemon over veal (and mushrooms) in pan. Stir all ingredients and continue to cook for 1–2 minutes more. Season with garlic powder, parsley, and paprika to taste.

1,200-Calorie Plan
1 serving veal piccata (5-ounce veal cutlet)

1,400-Calorie Plan
1 serving veal piccata (5-ounce veal cutlet)

Salad with lettuce, tomatoes, carrots, onion, peppers, and
mushrooms

2 tablespoons low-fat or nonfat Italian dressing

1,600-Calorie Plan

1 serving veal piccata (5-ounce veal cutlet)

Salad with lettuce, tomatoes, carrots, onion, peppers, and
mushrooms

2 tablespoons low-fat or nonfat Italian dressing

1/2 cup brown rice

LINGUINI AND WHITE CLAM SAUCE

Yields 6 1-cup servings.

3/4 pound linguini (12 ounces dry)

4 tablespoons olive oil

2 tablespoons jarred garlic, chopped

2 61/2-ounce cans of clams, minced or chopped

1 tablespoon lemon juice concentrate

1/2 cup white wine

Pepper to taste

4 tablespoons Parmesan cheese

Cook pasta as directed on box. While pasta is boiling, coat a frying
pan with olive oil and garlic. Cook and stir over low-medium flame
until lightly browned. Add clams (with clam juice), lemon juice,
wine, and pepper. Bring mixture back to a boil, lower heat, and

simmer for 3 minutes. Pour over drained pasta and mix thoroughly. Add Parmesan cheese and mix thoroughly.

1,200-Calorie Plan

1 cup linguini and white clam sauce

1,400-Calorie Plan

1 cup linguini and white clam sauce

Salad with lettuce, tomatoes, carrots, onion, peppers, and mushrooms

2 tablespoons low-fat or nonfat Italian dressing

1,600-Calorie Plan

1½ cups linguini and white clam sauce

½ cup steamed carrots or peapods or green beans

PORK TENDERLOIN
WITH CREAMY ZUCCHINI SOUP

PORK TENDERLOIN

Yields 4 servings.

2 tablespoons low-sodium soy sauce

¼ cup bourbon (or other liquor)

1 tablespoon brown sugar

1½ pounds pork tenderloin

¼ cup reduced-fat sour cream

¼ cup low-fat mayonnaise

1 tablespoon scallions

1 tablespoon dried mustard

1 tablespoon vinegar

Preheat oven to 325°F.

    To prepare marinade, mix soy sauce, liquor, and brown sugar. In a plastic bag, marinate pork tenderloin for 2–3 hours. Cook for 1 hour at 325°F.

    Make sauce by mixing sour cream, mayonnaise, scallions, mustard, and vinegar. Serve sauce on the side or pour over the pork tenderloin.

CREAMY ZUCCHINI SOUP

Yields 10 cups. (The remainder can be frozen for future meals.)

1 onion

2 teaspoons olive oil

3 pounds zucchini, peeled and sliced

1 potato, peeled and sliced

4 cups chicken broth

1 cup skim milk

In a large pan, sauté onion with olive oil until soft. Add sliced zucchini, potato, chicken broth, and milk. Cook over medium heat until soft. Pour entire mixture into food processor and purée.

1,200-Calorie Plan

1 piece of pork tenderloin with sauce (1/4 of prepared dish)

Sliced cucumber

1,400-Calorie Plan

1 piece of pork tenderloin with sauce (1/4 of prepared dish)

1 cup of creamy zucchini soup

1,600-Calorie Plan

1 piece of pork tenderloin with sauce (1/4 of prepared dish)

2 cups of creamy zucchini soup

Sliced cucumber

VEGETABLE COUSCOUS

Yields 2 servings.

1 cup cooked couscous

3/4 cup chickpeas

1 tablespoon olive oil

1 zucchini, peeled and diced

1 cup squash (any type), peeled and diced

Salt and pepper to taste

Garlic, fresh or powdered

1/2 cup crushed tomatoes, canned

3 tablespoons Parmesan cheese

Steam couscous in a pot as directed. Add chickpeas in couscous and set aside. In a frying pan, combine olive oil, zucchini, and squash. Add in salt, pepper, and garlic while stirring. As vegetables get soft, add in crushed tomatoes. Lower heat and simmer. Once tomato/vegetable combination is bubbling, pour into pot with couscous and chickpeas, and cook over low flame. Sprinkle on Parmesan cheese and mix thoroughly.

1,200-Calorie Plan
1/2 portion of vegetable couscous

1,400-Calorie Plan
1/2 portion of vegetable couscous
1 small, whole-wheat pita bread, toasted

1,600-Calorie Plan
1/2 portion of vegetable couscous
1 regular-sized, whole-wheat pita bread, toasted
1/2 grapefruit or 1 orange or 1 peach

Recipes are listed in boldface by category.

ABOUT THE AUTHOR

Joy Bauer, M.S., R.D., C.D.N. was named **Best Nutritionist in New York City** by *New York Magazine.* Recognized as one of the leading nutrition authorities, Joy maintains a thriving private practice where she provides counseling to both adults and children, dealing with a variety of nutritional concerns including weight management, diabetes, eating disorders, cardiac rehabilitation, sports nutrition, food allergies, gastrointestinal disorders, pregnancy, lactation, and menopause. Her clientele include high-profile professionals, and celebrity actors, models, and Olympic athletes.

An active speaker in her field, Joy regularly lectures throughout the United States and frequently appears on national television shows, including *Later Today, The View, Entertainment Tonight, TV Food Network,* and the *Fox News Channel.* She is regularly interviewed and featured in national publications, including *Fitness, Fit, Cosmopolitan, McCalls, Woman's Day, Women's Sports and Fitness, Marie Claire, Seventeen, Allure,* and the *New York Post.* Joy is also the author of *The Complete Idiot's Guide to Eating Smart* and its second edition, *The Complete Idiot's Guide to Total Nutrition.*

Joy received her bachelor's degree in kinesiological sciences from the University of Maryland and continued on to New York University to receive a Master of Science in nutrition. At the beginning of her career, Joy completed a five-year post as director of nutrition and fitness for the Heart-Smart Kids Program—a program that she developed for the Mount Sinai Medical Center in New York City's Department of Pediatric Cardiology.

She was the primary nutrition consultant to Columbia Presbyterian Medical Center in New York City, where she designed and supervised their ongoing research in the area of eating disorders and weight management, and has served as a clinical nutritionist with the neurosurgical team at Mount Sinai Medical Center.

In addition, Joy has instructed classes in anatomy and physiology, and sports nutrition at New York University's School of Continuing Education, and was the exclusive nutritionist for New York University's faculty, students, and athletes.

Joy lives in New York with her husband, Ian; her daughters, Jesse and Ayden; and her son, Cole.

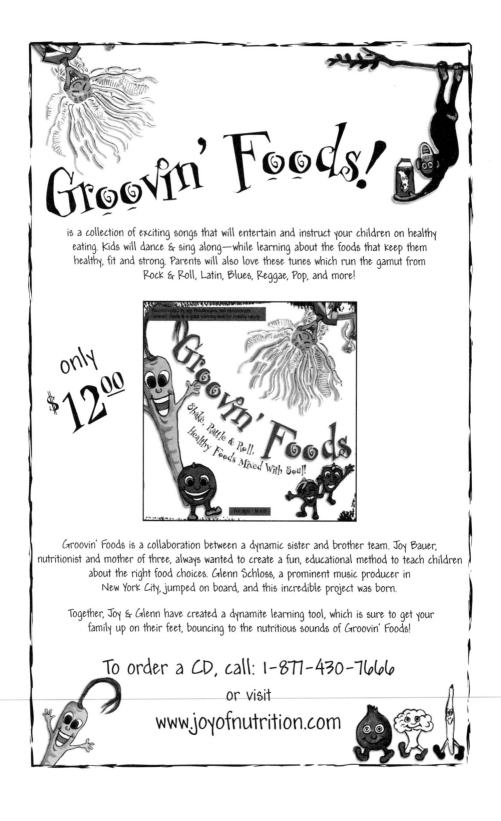